Resistance Band Exercises for Seniors Over 50

2 Books in 1 – Simple Workouts to Build Strength, Energy, Mobility, and Stability

Francis Papun

Book 1: Resistance Band Workouts

Table of Contents

Book 2: Bodyweight Workouts

Table of Contents

Introduction

"Aging is not lost youth, but a new stage of opportunity and strength." — Betty Friedan, Author and Activist

Sarah was telling her friends about her attempt at exercising at the age of 68. "I got permission from my doctor to join the fitness group. The first time I jumped, gyrated, huffed, and puffed for over an hour. By the time I got my leotard on, it was past the class's starting time!"

Fitness and mobility do not have to be such elusive goals for seniors. It may seem hard to believe that anyone battling decreasing suppleness and lamenting their level of fitness can maintain a routine the same as when they were younger.

Is getting up in the morning harder than it used to be? Are your joints achy and stiff, and is bending down to pick something up a major issue? Are you afraid of going downstairs because you don't feel confident in your balance? Does your list of chronic medications keep getting longer?

Do you suffer from anxiety attacks and depression because you fear losing your independence and mobility? Do you miss the overall good feeling of having exercised your body and being rid of all the creaks and pains that sometimes seem to appear overnight?

If the idea of going to a gym to get moving again is even scarier than the possible consequences of doing no exercise at all, this book is here to help. Packed full of information about training without risk of injury while maximizing strength and therapeutic benefits, and staying in your own home to boot, the book is a treasure trove of helpful exercises. You will see how easy it is to get your fitness and health back with only minimal equipment required, and objects already in your home. It is simple and economical - an elegant solution to a health problem.

The information can be taken with you wherever you travel, so you never have to miss any training session on account of being in a hotel or on vacation. Resistance bands are lightweight and compact and you will learn how to choose your purchases wisely to make a wide variety of exercises possible with only a few different bands.

Each exercise has been discussed in detail and all care was taken to describe them as plainly as possible. Most of the exercises have been adapted to standing or sitting positions. Skip those that have to be done lying down on the floor especially if your body is not comfortable in this position, or try to modify them for more comfortable surfaces to lie on. While your workout should challenge you, it should never be painful; listen to your body to achieve the best results. You should not exercise to the point of collapsing after the last repetition.

Be sure to consult your physician before starting the program. This is especially true for anyone who has not trained in a while. If you are worried about the possible effects on any old injury you might be nursing or any existing medical conditions, obtain an expert's opinion first and put your mind at rest. Physiotherapists and personal trainers experienced in injury rehabilitation will be able to evaluate any exercise and see possible warning signs to prevent damage. Sometimes just a small modification to a movement might be all that's needed to make it safe for you and help you obtain the full benefit of your training program.

Your mental attitude will make a big difference in the success of any training program. Worries about hurting yourself will hold you back from achieving the results that are possible with the training routines in this book.

How Will This Book Benefit Me?

These simple but powerful explanations and practical applications will make it easy to assess your unique fitness needs and design an exercise routine to suit any requirements. The versatility of resistance bands makes them an ideal exercise tool. They are lightweight and compact, making them easy to transport. They can be used in- or outdoors, at home or on vacation.

You will learn about the various types of tubing and bands available and how to choose the ideal one for you. You will also learn how to use the equipment correctly to prevent strain injuries, stay toned and fit, keep blood pressure normal, and aid in the healing of any existing injuries or post medical procedures.

Armed with information about the different body types, you will be able to put together a set of exercises tailored for your age, fitness level, and specific training for an activity or sport.

Who Is the Author?

Francis Papun is an ardent fitness enthusiast and coach who has helped individuals the last two decades take back control over their health and fitness. He is passionate about helping people build perfect bodies and healthier minds.

He believes in continual development and strives to assist people who want to achieve their happiest lives. Inspiring the youth to devote enough time to nurture healthy, strong bodies is also an important belief. He has a genuine desire to help others and knows success is only possible through dedication and hard work.

An author of a variety of health and fitness topics, Francis's aim is to help the reader understand staying fit and agile is not as hard as it seems. His books explain the secrets to making the necessary lifestyle changes that will transform body and mind. He leverages health and fitness training to polish and hone all the key attributes of people who struggle to keep up with a fast-moving world.

Francis is an expert at building robust fitness plans and aims to amalgamate his extensive knowledge and passion for fitness to help his readers to build perfect versions of themselves.

Besides this, Francis Papun remains an avid seeker of knowledge. He is always on the lookout for something new to learn, as well as staying alert to every opportunity to make a positive difference in someone's life.

He cherishes his family and friends and loves spending time with them.

Benefits of Regular Exercise for Seniors

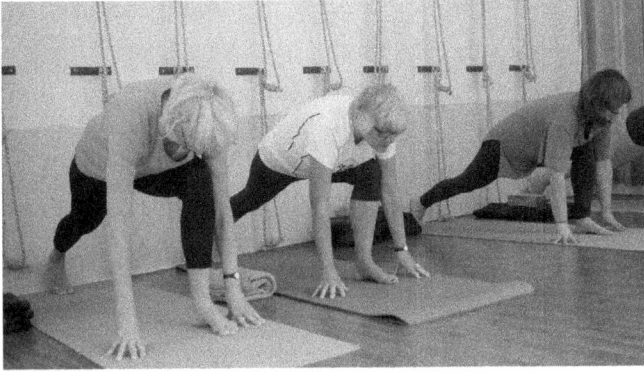

A moving body is a healthy body, even well into old age. Regular exercise of the right kind has numerous benefits.

Prevention of Disease

Heart disease, hypertension, and diabetes have become part of our daily existence, and some people believe that contracting these illnesses in advanced years is unavoidable.

Regular exercise, however, strengthens the heart muscle, lowers blood pressure, and raises the levels of good cholesterol. This brings about better blood flow throughout the body and ensures more efficient heart activity ("Health Benefits of Physical Activity," 2019).

Weight Management

Excess weight is a well-known risk factor in many diseases. Regular exercise increases the body's ability to burn calories and builds muscle mass for a stronger, healthier body.

Pain Management

Back pain is a common complaint among seniors. If it is caused by weak muscles that can no longer properly support the bone structure, regular exercise targeted at the right muscle groups will improve posture and add flexibility, thereby preventing or lessening back pain ("Health Benefits of Physical Activity," 2019).

Bone Health

The condition of osteoporosis refers to fragile bones. When the formation of new bone cannot keep up with the loss of the old tissue, the bone structure becomes stressed. This weakens them to the point where even mild accidents can cause bone fractures. Regular strengthening exercises can prevent this from happening and minimize risk in older people. Women are especially prone to osteoporosis after menopause (Mayo Clinic, 2016).

Stress Reduction

Many studies have shown that physical exercise leads to an increase in mood-regulating chemicals (Collins, 2012). Movement stimulates inactive parts of the brain and neurotransmitters such as dopamine, serotonin, and endorphins are released. That also helps to maintain a balance with stress hormones such as adrenalin.

Prevention of Disability

Flexible, strong joints and muscles are an excellent defense against falls or accidents. It lowers the risk of serious injury and consequent disability significantly.

Maintaining Cognitive Function

Regular exercise has been shown to lower the risk of dementia by about 30 percent. Some studies suggest the risk for specifically Alzheimer's disease could even be halved when an exercise routine is started in later life (Alzheimer's Society UK, n.d.).

Social Engagement

A regular workout routine shared with others can provide essential social contact for seniors. Feelings of loneliness won't stand a chance, and exercising will never feel like a chore again.

My Promise to You

If you apply the easy principles explained in this book and invest time in compiling and regularly performing a set of resistance band exercises tailored to your needs, guided by the detailed information in this book, your body will yield years of interest on your investment.

You will experience far greater flexibility and fitness, as well as a much higher level of health than your peers who opted for inactivity. You will have the opportunity to prevent or improve some serious and debilitating illnesses.

The benefits are long-lasting because each exercise routine can easily be adjusted according to evolving needs. With portable and lightweight equipment like resistance bands, exercise can carry on well into advanced age.

But...You Have to Act!

There is no better time than the present to take control of your health and quality of life. You have all the tools you need in your hands with this book, regardless of your current age. Stop merely surviving and start thriving. Let's get started!

Chapter 1: What is Resistance Training?

According to its definition, resistance, or strength training is described as activities of any kind that make muscles stronger (Merriam-Webster, 2011).

When thinking about resistance training, the first image that's likely to pop into your head is of burly muscled athletes lifting weights and barbells. It does not have to be that way though. This type of training can be done with the aid of simple tools, or bodyweight alone can be used to provide resistance. Its effectiveness lies in the fact that it builds muscle strength and endurance.

How Exactly Does the Body Build Muscle?

The easiest way to explain the process is to think about damage and subsequent repair happening within the body. Skeletal muscles are some of the most adaptable tissue in the body, and they always strive to repair any injury to fibers as soon as possible. This is done by rebuilding the injured muscle through satellite cells, which fuse and adhere to the muscle fibers. This enlarges the muscle and is known as cell hypertrophy (Kwon & Kravitz, 2019).

It is necessary to understand the word injury in a broader sense. Exercising a muscle and challenging it to its limits with an activity like resistance training causes trauma to the fibers inside the muscle. This trauma is referred to as injury in scientific terms, although it does not necessarily involve pain in the traditional sense of the word (Kwon & Kravitz, 2019). It is also called micro-trauma (Creveling, 2020).

The newly added satellite cells provide additional growth nuclei to the muscle, which enables the muscle to synthesize more protein than before and also utilize these building blocks more effectively than before.

One of the biggest advantages of using body weight as resistance is that no unnecessary load is added (Creveling, 2020). That yields the biggest gains in strength and flexibility for everyday activities with the least damage done. A win-win situation!

Studies have also shown regular resistance exercise to increase the protecting tissue network around muscles, thereby reducing the risk of injury even more (Kwon & Kravitz, 2019).

Other ways to build strength are:

- Pull-ups
- Squats
- Push-ups
- Planking
- Burpees
- Tricep dips
- Crawls
- Mountain climbers
- Box jumps

None of these methods involve any weights.

Why Are Bands a Good Choice?

There are several reasons why resistance bands or resistance tubing are a good choice for seniors (Lori Michiel Fitness, Inc, n.d.). Resistance bands are small and easily folded into a compact space. That means they travel well and suit any lifestyle. The durable material means it can be used indoors and outdoors. All levels of fitness can benefit from this type of training. While some super athletes regularly include resistance training with bands in their routines, it works equally well for someone just starting out with a new program or recovering from an injury. No gravity pull is involved like with weights, making it a very safe form of exercise. Because the body has to be stabilized all the time to counter the tension while using resistance bands, it greatly enhances coordination and balance.

Bands can be used to perform new and basic moves, or they can be incorporated into an existing routine to add variety and intensity. Just by positioning your body relative to the band differently, a new group of muscles can be targeted with the same exercise (Lori Michiel Fitness, Inc, n.d.).

Bands can be purchased in different strengths, as well as different forms and sizes. There are flat models or those rounded with handles also known as tubing. Many of them are color-coded according to various tension levels from easy to very heavy. Pink and yellow generally mean light tension, green and red moderate, and dark gray and black are considered intense. Generally, resistance bands are cheaply priced, especially if you want to purchase only one first to get started and see if it works for you. They can be purchased in stores or online.

No specialized equipment or installation is necessary to reap the full benefits of resistance band training. They can be looped around the body or anchored to a chair or table, or simply be pinned to the floor by hands or feet.

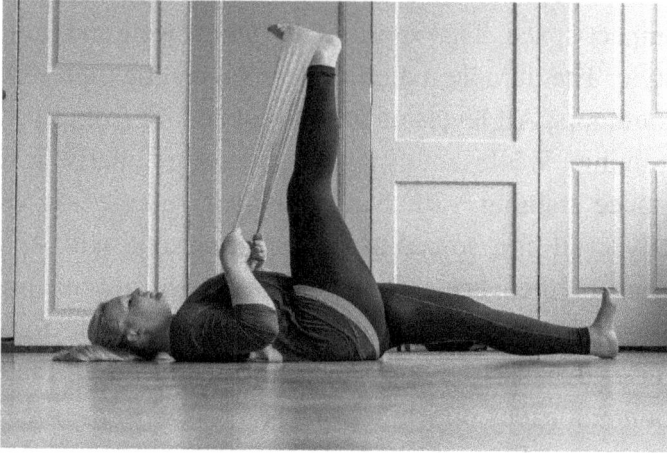

Flat band

Making the Right Choice

A good way to start is by buying a set of three or four coordinated mini-bands with different resistance levels. The standard circumference is between 18 and 24 inches.

Add a pull-up assistance band to assist with movement without having to use full body weight. This type of band is longer than the mini-bands and should be strong enough to withstand all the bodyweight of the individual using it.

Look for bands that are comfortable to use. Padded, permanent handles usually feel more comfortable than detachable plastic handles.

Make sure the equipment you buy has all the accessories needed to make it fully functional. And always check with your doctor first if you have any existing condition or injury.

The Top 10 Resistance Band Training Rules

As with any activity, following simple rules for your safety and comfort is the best way to make the most out of your training sessions and achieve lasting results.

- **Always warm-up and stretch**

Before beginning any exercise routine, it is extremely important to warm the muscles and joints slowly up first. This will also ensure heart rate and body temperature don't spike but build up gradually to a level where exercise can be performed safely.

At the end of the program, the body has to be stretched gently to cool down. That will give the cardiovascular system a chance to return to resting levels in a controlled way (*The Right Way to Warm Up and Cool Down*, 2019).

In one of the later chapters, we'll delve deeper into dynamic warm-ups and stretching exercises.

- **Start with 30-minute sessions**

It might be tempting to jump into your new exercise routine with so much gusto that you feel you could achieve everything within a month. However, that is setting yourself up for failure.

Start with a commitment of only 30 minutes at a time and increase the time slowly as your strength and fitness grow.

13

Once you are well-conditioned, the sessions can be continued up to 90 minutes.

- **Build a habit**

Muscle strength builds slowly, but it will only happen if training happens regularly. Sporadic training will decrease endurance and motivation, while the risk for injury is increased (YMCA of the North, n.d.).

- **Increase repetitions gradually**

A good number of repetitions to start with is eight. Gradually increase this to 15 and listen to your body to determine how quickly this can be done (Fitness Australia, 2018).

- **Aim for at least ten exercises**

Try to include ten exercises in your routine. Four of these should be for your lower body and six for the upper body. This should add enough variety to keep things interesting.

- **Perform movements in a controlled fashion**

Less really is more for seniors in terms of gains from exercise when controlled movements are used instead of power and momentum. A fast, strong movement targets different muscles than a slower, controlled one.

With the goals of balance and flexibility in mind, the muscles that control movement are the ones that should be exercised (Crowley, 2016).

- **Work larger muscles first**

As a general rule, larger muscles are exercised before smaller muscles (Jay, 2010). That means, for instance, working chest muscles first before getting to the shoulders. More difficult exercises will come before easier ones.

- **Perform a complete range of motion**

Performing the complete range of motion that a muscle is capable of, is the best way to exercise the whole muscle. This is especially important in the case of seniors, where regaining flexibility and mobility is vital. Using the full range of capabilities of a specific muscle will alleviate stiffness and pain caused by limited movements (Fetters, 2016).

It should be a pain-free movement, continuing as far as the joint will allow. Adjust the amount of resistance to accommodate a full range of motion.

- **Never hold your breath**

Correct breathing is very important and will be discussed in a later chapter. It is easy when concentrating on movement or form to hold your breath, as counterintuitive as that may sound.

Because our bodies are smart, our brains know when muscles need more oxygen. Oxygen is delivered in blood, so the heart rate increases to meet the higher demand. Holding your breath can cause your blood pressure to rise, due to the lack of adequate oxygen. This will achieve exactly the opposite result of what you want (Alexander, 2011). Instead, use the rhythm of exercise to learn deep and calm breathing.

- **Maintain the correct body alignment**

Body alignment or exercise posture refers to the relative positions of different body parts to each other during an exercise. Ignoring this can lead to injury or aggravate an existing condition.

General guidelines to keep in mind are (National Posture Institute, 2014):

- The head should be kept in line with the spine as far as possible, positioning the ears over the shoulders.
- The chin should be in line with the neck.
- The back should be straight, and the shoulders relaxed.
- The knees should not be locked.
- The pelvis should be tucked in somewhat, with the belly button pushing towards the spine.

When progressing too quickly to a more difficult exercise or higher resistance before the body is ready, muscles and joints will compensate for their difficulty in performing the movement by going out of alignment. That can put your whole exercise routine on hold for quite a while and cause unnecessary pain and discomfort.

The Bottom Line

Are you excited yet about the new you that is only one resistance band away? Seriously, the benefits of resistance band training almost speak for themselves.

Let's summarize the main takeaways of this chapter:

- Resistance training does not automatically equal extra weights. Although weightlifting is probably the best-known form of strength exercise, the same results can be achieved with resistance bands only.
- Strength training works because of the way our bodies build new muscle.
- Resistance bands are an excellent choice for seniors specifically because they are versatile, portable, light, cheap, easily obtainable, easy to use, and they enhance coordination, flexibility, and balance more than other types of strength training.
- If you follow the ten rules of resistance band training and you have the go-ahead from your physician, it is one of the safest forms of exercise possible for seniors. Just to recap:
  - Always do warm-ups before and stretches after exercising.
  - Stick to half an hour sessions for a start.
  - Make it a habit.
  - Increase repetitions gradually.
  - Work up to ten exercises per session.
  - Control movements.
  - Work on larger muscles first.
  - Perform the full range of motion a muscle can do.
  - Breathe!
  - Keep proper body alignment.

In only a few weeks' time, you will feel supercharged and people will start to notice your confidence and radiance.

So get started today, why wait?

Chapter 2: Healing From Injury

Training with resistance bands to recuperate from an injury is an excellent way to strengthen the muscles again after a period of inactivity.

As with any exercise activity, seniors should keep a few things in mind when embarking on this healing journey to make it effective and prevent aggravation of the injury.

Common Injuries Healed With Resistance Training

Resistance bands are the ideal aids to focus on the muscle or group of damaged muscles because the maximum amount of stress can be put on the muscle without straining the joint unduly (*Rehabbing Sports Injuries with Resistance Bands*, 2018).

Shoulder Dislocation or Pain

According to a study done by the American Academy of Orthopaedic Surgeons, about one-fifth of all shoulder dislocations occur in patients older than 60 years. These patients are also more likely to suffer injury to the rotator cuff during dislocation because the tissue surrounding the cuff gets weaker with age (Murthi & Ramirez, 2012).

Older populations the world over are more active for longer than a few decades ago, and injuries can occur easily.

Other signs to watch for without actual dislocation having taken place are tingling or numbness, significant weakening of the hand and arm when compared to the other side, and persistent and unexplained pain or tenderness in the area.

Tennis Elbow

Contrary to popular belief, tennis elbow does not only come from prolonged tennis play. Any repetitive motion that damages the tendons connecting the forearm to the elbow can cause pain in the outer part of the elbow.

Activities such as gardening, painting, using a screwdriver, or even knitting or crocheting can be the source of the damage. The main concept here is overuse (Healthwise Incorporated, 2020).

Any rehab exercises should aim to lengthen the tendons again and strengthen them.

Runner's Knee

Another slight misnomer, the condition does not refer to a specific injury. It is a term that is used to indicate a broad range of knee problems, and the medical term is patellofemoral pain syndrome (WebMD, 2007).

It can be caused by any repetitive movement, for which the knee is not strong enough like stepping up the number of repetitions in an exercise routine too soon, or by a fall or other direct hit to the kneecap. Misalignment between hips and ankles or thigh muscles that are too weak to keep the kneecap in its proper place during movement could also cause pain, as can any foot problems common in the elderly (WebMD, 2007).

Hip Bursitis

Large joints like hips have fluid-filled sacs called bursae next to them to lubricate movement and protect the bone. If a bursae becomes inflamed for any reason, the condition is called bursitis.

Overuse, injury, or complications after hip surgery can cause it. Poor posture and weak muscles could predispose a person to develop bursitis (WebMD, n.d.).

Sprains and Strains

These two types of injuries have proved to be the nemesis of many older athletes. A resistance band workout offers a safe way to build strength again slowly.

A sprain occurs when a ligament is overstretched or overworked, while a strain refers to the same mechanism injuring a muscle or tendon (Giacobbe, 2019).

As soon as the injury has healed enough to allow for exercising, resistance bands for easy stretching can be used to gradually get moving again. As strength returns, bands with higher tension can be introduced until the ligament, muscle or tendon is back to the pre-injury level.

Recovery After Knee-Repair Surgery

This type of surgery is usually performed to repair the anterior cruciate ligaments or ACL. These ligaments hold the knee together and can get injured by a movement as simple as getting out of a car and turning too quickly to another direction.

In older people, the injury is often associated with weakened hamstrings (Quinn, 2020). Resistance band exercises present the perfect opportunity to strengthen and lengthen the hamstrings again gradually while also strengthening the knee and surrounding ligaments themselves.

Phases of Recuperation After Injury

Understanding the general phases of recovery can be very helpful in designing the right post-injury exercise routine. Three stadia can be identified as (New Heights Physical Therapy, n.d.):

- Reaction
- Regeneration
- Remodeling

Reaction Phase

The first 24 to 72 hours after sustaining an injury, the body responds to the trauma with swelling and muscle spasms among other things. Movement is painful and the natural reaction to this is to take painkillers and immobilize the injured part of the body.

A small, controlled amount of movement is necessary, however, to aid in the flushing of waste products and bringing in much-needed oxygen and nutrients to prevent the formation of scar tissue and start the healing process (New Heights Physical Therapy, n.d.).

Regeneration

The formation of new tissue and the repair of any damaged nerve connections starts next and takes anywhere between six and eight weeks (New Heights Physical Therapy, n.d.).

The aim of any physical exercise during this period is to minimize pain while maximizing the generation and strengthening of new tissue. One of the ways to do this is to gently increase the range of motion in a controlled manner.

Remodeling Stage

This is the final stage to complete recovery and can take between three months to a year. Although acute pain might be something of the past by now, it is still extremely important to manage the exercise routine correctly to prevent chronic pain from developing.

The focus should be on strengthening supporting tissue, muscles, and ligaments because the area is vulnerable and there is a danger of recurring injury (New Heights Physical Therapy, n.d.).

A Note of Caution

No workout should be started without consulting your physician first, especially not when recovering from an injury.

Be cautious if you:

- Have any shortness of breath without exertion.
- Have chest pains or pain in your left arm and neck.
- Take medication for high blood pressure.

- Have arthritis.
- Have osteoporosis.
- Have dizzy spells.
- Are extremely overweight.
- Have diabetes.

Always make sure you listen to your body. A good rule of thumb to follow is the "talk test." You should be able to talk normally while exercising. If you get out of breath, it is time to take it slower (Schrift, 2014).

Breathe, Breathe, Breathe...

Breathing is one of those automatic, instinctive actions needed for our survival, and it might sound strange to be reminded to do it. Many people, however, when they exercise, forget to breathe or breathe incorrectly during a movement.

Muscles use more oxygen when contracting than when resting, and the only way to deliver the much-needed element is by breathing deeply in the right pattern.

In and Out

The simplest breathing technique is to breathe in on a contraction and out on an extension (Taraniuk, 2019).

Let's illustrate that with some easy exercises:

- Squat: Breathe in while lowering your body into a squatting position (contraction). Breathe out while straightening your legs to a standing position again (extension).

- Chest press: Exhale as you push the resistance band handles away from you, inhale as you bring your hands back toward your chest.
- Glute bridge: Exhale when lifting your hips off the floor and inhale when lowering them again.

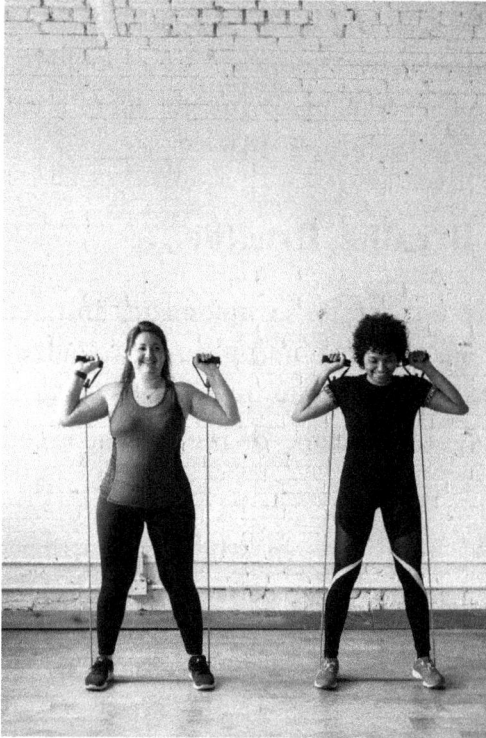

Women with flexible bands, ready to do a chest press

Belly Breathing

It is deeper than chest breathing and is also called diaphragmatic breathing. When you pull air in through your nose and feel your belly puffing up, you are using your diaphragm.

Benefits of belly breathing include lowering of heart rate and blood pressure, as well as enhancing the body's capacity for enduring exercise (Jewell, 2018).

A good way to teach yourself belly breathing is to concentrate on a sequence of breathing in for three counts and breathing out for two (Newhouse, 2013). If you do this while going about everyday activities, it will be second nature when you start your workout routine.

Consistency Is Key

Whether you do your workout three times a week or five times a week, being consistent matters more than the type of exercises or number of repetitions in terms of measurable results.

In a recent study undertaken by the University of New South Wales in Sydney's School of Medical Sciences, lead author Mandy Hagstrom found consistent and frequent exercise to be some of the key factors in a successful resistance training program (Hagstrom et al., 2019).

It is therefore important to set realistic goals for yourself. Design your workout to fit into your daily and monthly schedule. Make allowances for any illnesses or physical weaknesses you might have. Unrealistic goals lead to unrealistic expectations, which set you up for failure before you've even started.

Your health and well-being are far too important to sabotage your success by aiming too high.

The Role of Genetics

Our genes are the inescapable blueprints of who we are. They determine everything, from hair and eye color to personality.

Genes also determine body type, which influences how easy or difficult it is to get fit and flexible. But being inescapable does not equal the end of workout plans if your body type, it just means you may have to work a bit smarter to gain the same results as someone else.

The concept of different general body types has been around since the time of Plato. In the 1940s, American psychologist William Sheldon popularized three categories here (Snape, 2015) and identified them as ectomorph, endomorph, and mesomorph.

Each type has to train differently from the others, because muscle composition, among other factors, seems to vary.

Ectomorphs

This body type, especially among women, is very envied in modern times because they are skinny, long-limbed people who never seem to gain weight. They have fast metabolisms that rapidly convert sugars into energy.

This is not without problems though, because they have to work much harder to gain muscle mass through exercise. This has consequences in later years when muscle mass starts decreasing with age, and an exercise routine for a senior ectomorph will look different from any of the others.

Endomorphs

These are the bigger, pear-shaped people with shorter limbs and broader hips. They tend to put on weight easily. Unfortunately, a lot of this weight is fat and not muscle. They often have the hardest time getting fit and toned, but it is definitely attainable.

Ectomorphs

This group seems to fall in the middle of the first two. They don't store fat as easily and don't find it too hard to build muscle.

They are often referred to as "naturally athletic," and chances are that fitness was neglected in their younger days because they did not seem to need to workout.

The later years bring their own challenges with diminishing muscle mass and declining mobility, so this body type can benefit just as much from a regular resistance band routine as any of the others.

Types of Resistance Bands

There are six types of bands, and some have very specific uses. They are mini bands (also known as fit loop bands), tubing, therapy bands, figure 8 bands, ring bands, and lateral resistance bands.

The first two are the most versatile for general purposes (*The Definitive Guide to Resistance Bands and Workout Bands*, n.d.).

Mini Bands

They are flat with no handles and form a continuous loop. They are generally four inches to two feet long, and although they work well to train the lower body, any muscle group can be targeted depending on the size of the band. They are ideal for reaching muscles that would otherwise be difficult to isolate.

Mini bands come in different widths, from paper-thin to thick, and can be made from a variety of materials. Latex is the most common type, but for those with a latex allergy, there are fabric and elastic types.

If you plan on buying only one type of band to start, mini bands are a good option. Go for a thicker version to allow for a wide scope of exercises.

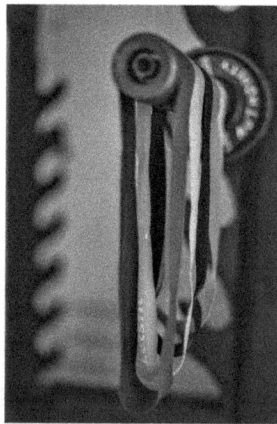

A set of mini bands

Tubing

These are tubular rather than flat as the title suggests, open-ended, and have handles at the ends. With an average length of around four feet, they are mostly used to strengthen the upper body.

Tubular bands are commonly found in gyms, personal training studios, and outdoor boot camps. Some have hooks attached to the ends so that different bands can be hooked together or other accessories can be attached.

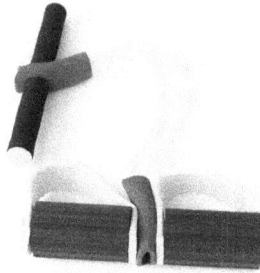

Tubular resistance band with handles

The Resistance Level

The intensity of a workout depends on the thickness of the band, as well as how far it is stretched. As you get stronger, you might decide not to change your exercises, but only to change the resistance before moving on to another exercise all together.

How to Find the Right Level

The appropriate resistance level at any given time depends on the exercise and the number of repetitions you're aiming for.

Start with the band offering the least resistance. The average number of repetitions should be between 10 and 15 for every exercise. You should feel challenged by about the seventh repetition. If you can do all the repetitions with this band without feeling tired, you should move up to the next band level (Kassel, 2019).

On the other hand, if you get the feeling during an exercise that you can't control the band, as if your arm or leg is about to be snapped back, then the resistance level is too high. Performing an exercise that way puts your body at risk of going out of alignment, which can be detrimental in the long run.

Adjusting Resistance During an Exercise

It is quick and simple to adjust on the go because resistance bands are so versatile.

You could either add bands, adjust your position or the position of the band.

- Adding bands to the one already in use will immediately increase the resistance experienced and make the exercise harder.
- Resistance is also influenced by the distance you stand from an anchor point in exercises that require anchors. For a standing row exercise, for example, the band needs to be looped around or fastened to an immovable object. Standing closer to the anchor point will make the exercise easier while moving away will make it harder.
- The resistance will change from a band looped above your knees to around your shins, then ankles.

Do You Need More Convincing?

If you're still wondering if resistance bands will work for you, let's look at the benefits again. The great thing is, these benefits will be accurate for you regardless of your age or fitness level (8fit Team, n.d.).

Resistance band workouts force muscles to contract when the band is stretched, which tones and strengthens. It is a controllable and gentle way for older people to achieve results. Resistance bands can also be used to assist in exercise. If a pull up for instance looks impossible to do, use a band attached to the bar to make it easier until you can perform it unassisted.

Nobody likes aching muscles, rigid and tight with tension. Use resistance bands to gently stretch back, shoulder, and neck muscles to remove the caught-up tension and find natural pain relief.

Your resistance bands will travel wherever you go. They're light and easy to fold, taking up very little space in a suitcase. As far as training equipment goes, this is one of the most affordable options available. The grandkids might even enjoy exercising with you!

Resistance bands don't need gravity to do their job like weights, which make them easier on joints and muscles that are not so young anymore. A wider range of motion is possible, which means better flexibility and strengthening can be achieved. Many exercises can be done in a sitting position, making an exercise routine accessible to people who might normally have been excluded.

Not only muscles but bones and joints benefit from resistance band workouts. Strength training stimulates bones to make new cells, keeping osteoporosis at bay and decreasing the likelihood of broken bones if a small tumble should happen.

The low impact of resistance band exercises is very kind to joints as well. They are also ideal for recovering after an injury when exercise should be targeted but gentle.

Before we start with the nitty-gritty of an exercise routine in the next chapters, this could be a good time to go back over the previous chapters and make sure you know and understand everything involved.

You can always refer back to this outline, and you might even pick something up that you missed the first time.

Are you ready to start warming up?

Chapter 3: Warm-Ups and Stretches

You wouldn't expect to be able to reach down to the floor and touch your toes first thing in the morning after getting out of bed stiffly and cautiously. Equally, you can't expect your body to perform exercise routines without having been prepared first.

Not only will muscles and joints be endangered if a proper warm-up is neglected, but to burst into sudden vigorous activity can overwork the heart. Warming up gradually speeds up the heart and breathing gradually, which delivers more blood and oxygen to the muscles and prepares them for more intense activity.

The reverse is true at the end of the workout if movement comes to a stop without gently slowing down with stretches. A cooling down stretching routine brings everything back to resting tempo with no sudden changes.

Furthermore, easing into your workout with warm-ups puts you in the right frame of mind to make the most of your active time.

Suggested Exercises

Let's look at a couple of warm-up exercises and stretches in practical detail.

Windmill Exercise

This exercise loosens the shoulders but is also very beneficial for core strength and overall stability (Fetters, 2019).

- Start by standing with your feet slightly wider than hip-width. Turn your left foot out at an angle of 90 degrees and raise your right arm to the ceiling while looking up at your right hand.
- Slide your left arm down your left leg as far as possible without putting any pressure on the leg. Bend the leg slightly to avoid locking the knee.
- Move your hips slightly to your right and use your core to stabilize yourself while sliding your left arm down.
- Pause at the lowest point for a couple of seconds before pushing yourself upright again. Keep your spine straight all the time.
- Do five to eight repetitions before switching sides.

Elbow Touch

This exercise is beneficial to the chest, shoulders, and rotator cuff.

- Sit or stand with proper body alignment and place your right hand on your right shoulder and your left hand on your left shoulder.
- Move your arms towards each other until your elbows touch.
- Move your elbows out to the sides while attempting to squeeze your shoulder blades closer to each other.
- Visualize your chest opening up and stretching to admit more oxygen.
- Return your elbows to the starting position in a controlled movement.
- Do five to eight repetitions.

Tennis Elbow Warm-Up

If you are exercising to help heal a tennis elbow, it is especially important to warm the elbow and surrounding muscles and tendons up first to avoid increasing pain.

- Sit at a table with your arm comfortably stretched out on the table, palm facing up.
- Touch every finger to your thumb, starting with the pinkie.
- Do five to eight repetitions before switching sides.

Shoulder Box Exercise

The target of this exercise is the trapezius muscle. It is a large triangular muscle in the upper back that stretches the whole width between the shoulders. It reaches down to the thoracic part of the spine (De Pietro, 2019).

The trapezius plays a big role in shoulder and neck mobility and helps to stabilize the shoulders during some arm movements.

Pain in this area is often caused by stress, overuse, or poor posture, such as sitting hunched over a computer all day.

- Tie your resistance band to a solid anchoring object at your shoulder height.
- Hold your arms straight out in front of you, level with your shoulders.
- Keep a little bit of tension in the band so that your chest pulls forward slightly.
- Move your arms out to the sides with the backs of your hands facing up.

- Squeeze your shoulders together for a couple of seconds before returning to the starting position slowly.
- Do five to eight repetitions (Mirafit, n.d.).

A variation without the resistance band can be done by standing comfortably with your arms hanging by your sides.

- While inhaling through the nose, slowly pull your shoulders up towards your ears, as far as is comfortable for you.
- Pull your shoulder blades back towards each other, and push your shoulders down at the same time.
- Hold for a couple of seconds before slowly returning to the starting position (Knopf, 2010).

Choker Exercise

The shoulders and rotator cuff are sometimes difficult to isolate and reach. This exercise is excellent for doing just that and is a great pain reliever when stress is the culprit.

- Sit or stand with your right hand on your left shoulder.
- Place your left hand under your right elbow and gently push your right arm upwards towards your throat so that your elbow stops in line with your nose.
- Hold for 10 seconds and release.
- Do five to eight repetitions and switch sides (Knopf, 2010).

A variation on this exercise for even more stretch is to take your right hand off your shoulder and straighten the arm when it reaches the top position.

Wrist Stretch

If you are a constant computer or smartphone user, your wrists will need special attention with a couple different stretches.

- Stretch your arm out in front of you with the palm turned up towards the ceiling.
- Bend your wrist down as far as possible so that your fingers point towards the floor.
- Take hold of your fingers with your other hand and gently pull them towards your body until you can feel a stretch in the underside of your wrist.
- Hold for a couple of seconds and relax.
- Repeat five to eight times.

Stretch the top of your wrist as well by doing the same exercise, only keep your palm facing the floor (Fort Healthcare, 2019).

Knee to Chest Exercise

The lower back and gluteus maximus (or glute for short) are often problem areas in older people. Glutes are the main hip muscles and are connected to the lower back and thighs. Spasms in this muscle can make it painful to stand up or sit down.

A comfortable and safe way to perform the knee to chest stretch is to do it in a prone position.

- Lie down fully stretched out on your back.
- Bring one knee up to your chest and wrap your arms around your leg below the knee.

- Pull the knee closer gently as far as is comfortable and hold for a couple of seconds.
- Lower the leg and do the same stretch with the other one.
- Repeat five to eight times.

If your back is strong enough, you could lift both knees at the same time (Kendola, 2020).

Sit & Reach Exercise

The next body parts to receive attention are the hamstrings. They are often shortened, stiff, and painful in seniors because of decreased mobility.

The sit and reach exercise is commonly used by fitness coaches to determine a person's flexibility and assess their risk for future injury.

- If it is possible for you, sit flat on the floor near a wall or other flat object, with your legs stretched out in front of you.
- Keep your knees straight and make sure feet are up against the wall while you remain flat on the floor.
- Bend forward and stretch your arms out as far as they can go.
- Keep the position for a couple of seconds.
- Repeat five times if possible (Quinn, 2008).

If you cannot sit on the floor, you can perform the exercise on a chair.

- Sit forward on the seat with one leg stretched out straight in front of you.

- Tilt the foot of the outstretched leg up.
- Bend forward, keeping your body in a straight line, and reach down with your hand towards your foot, as far as you can go.

Rear Calf Stretch Exercise

Tight or painful calves can hamper movement significantly. For the elderly, poor circulation is often to blame for this condition. This stretch can go a long way to alleviate the discomfort.

- Stand while holding on to the back of a chair with one foot in front of the other.
- Bend the knee of the front foot slightly.
- Lean forward towards the chair while keeping the back leg completely straight (Marcin, 2018).

Gas Pedal Exercise

Ankles are vulnerable and easy to injure when flexibility lessens, and movement becomes more difficult. It is, therefore, imperative to look after ankle health and make sure they are properly warmed up and stretched.

The gas pedal stretch is done with the aid of a resistance band.

- Sit on a chair with one leg stretched out in front of you and your back kept straight.
- Loop the band under the outstretched foot where the instep is.
- Pull the band up tight enough that you can feel tension around your foot.

- Push your foot down against the band as if you are using the gas pedal of a car.
- Repeat five to eight times and change feet (University Orthopedics, n.d.).

Twister Exercise

The torso twist is a great way to warm up your core muscles and enhance flexibility at the same time. A word of caution if you are prone to dizzy spells: take it slowly and carefully.

- Stand with your feet shoulder-width apart.
- Bend your elbows so your arms form a 90-degree angle.
- Swing your shoulders and torso from one side to the other.
- Look in the direction where you are moving and pivot your feet with the movement.
- Allow your right heel to lift when twisting to the left and the left heel to lift when twisting to the right.
- Keep your head up, and your neck relaxed.
- Remember to control the movement; don't jerk or try to do it too fast (Pedemonte, 2020).

Side Bend Exercise

Another good movement to benefit the torso and shoulders is the side bend.

- Stand with your feet comfortably placed about shoulder-width apart.
- Keep your back straight and bend down to one side, reaching with that hand towards the floor.

- Hold the stretch for a couple of seconds and come up slowly.
- Do the same to the other side.
- Remember to control the movement at all times so as not to compromise the spine (Winderl, 2017).

Rock 'n Roll Exercise

A slow, gentle version of rocking and rolling can do wonders for any tight or sore lower back area while strengthening the torso and core muscles.

- Lie down on your back on the floor.
- Pull your knees up and keep your feet flat on the ground.
- Roll your knees slowly and gently to one side and then to the other.
- Make sure your shoulders stay firmly on the ground and don't move with your lower body.
- Repeat five to eight times (Cadman, 2020).

Head Lift Exercise

A stiff and painful neck is, unfortunately, one of the realities of our modern, stressful life. It is also a vulnerable part of the body and should be warmed up gently to prevent injury.

- Go down on your hands and knees and keep your body in alignment with hands under shoulders and knees under hips.
- Keep your back straight and drop your head slowly down towards your chest.
- Tuck in your chin and hold the position for five seconds.

- Then raise your head again slowly to be level with your back.
- Do five to eight repetitions.
- Remember to keep the movement controlled at all times (Fairview, n.d.).

Tennis Watcher Exercise

Another one for the neck is done seated.

- Inhale through your nose and look towards your left as far as you can comfortably turn your head.
- Hold the position for a few seconds.
- Exhale through your mouth, and slowly turn your head back to face forwards again.
- Repeat the process to the other side.
- Keep the movement slow and controlled.
- Do five to eight repetitions (Dotfit, n.d.).

Chapter 4: Understanding the Benefits of Strength Training

Every journey has to start somewhere. Deciding to exercise towards a healthier, fitter, and happier you is no exception.

You might have tried in the past only to be turned around or mitigated some of the negative consequences of getting older. Anything new can be scary and uncomfortable at first, especially if you are not fully convinced you will make a difference.

If you are still on the fence about strength training, I want to tell you a bit more about this concept and its benefits for you. I understand your hesitation and would like to show you where this can lead if you allow it to keep building momentum.

Strength Training in a Nutshell

Strength or resistance training helps muscles and joints remain fully functional at any age, and preserves mobility well into the golden years. Strong, flexible muscles and joints make daily activities much easier and contribute to general happiness and a feeling of well-being. Workouts can be adapted to all fitness levels, and most existing chronic diseases can be managed and even improved through regular resistance training sessions (Mayo Clinic, 2018). Let's break this down into more bite-size chunks.

From the age of 30, we start losing muscle mass to the tune of three to five percent per year (Iliades, 2019). Strength workouts can be designed with exercises that target specific muscles or muscle groups, making them stronger and stimulating them to form new tissue.

If a muscle has a problem already like the back, strengthening the muscles around the problem area minimizes pain and discomfort and makes movement easier. Stronger muscles protect the joints around which they are, so the joints can keep functioning the way they should (Iliades, 2019).

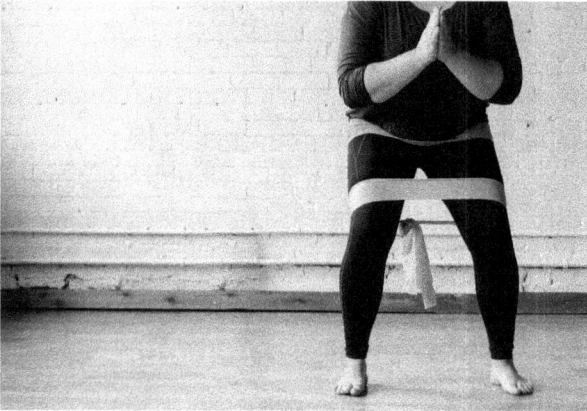

Exercise stimulates the cells that form new bone. That will prevent osteoporosis, which is the weakening of bones mostly in older people. If there is osteoporosis already present, the condition will improve when bone density increases. The hips, spine, and wrists are prime candidates for osteoporosis and will benefit greatly from strength training (Wheeler, 2019).

Many seniors complain of struggling to keep their balance. Everyday things like climbing stairs become a nightmare, which has a limiting effect on their enjoyment of life. The balance problem stems from weakness in the hips, legs, ankles, and all the surrounding muscles. The right resistance exercises target these areas and restore strength. That decreases the likelihood of falls and fractures, which boosts self-confidence and quality of life (Wheeler, 2019).

A strength workout with resistance bands eliminates the need to visit a gym to gain access to equipment and personal trainers. You already have everything you need to make the most out of the bands in your home. With this book in your hands, there are no more excuses to get started.

Physical exercise is an instant mood boost. The exertion causes dopamine and other feel good neurotransmitters to be released in the brain, which brings feelings of happiness and a relaxed frame of mind. A regular resistance workout burns calories and helps to keep weight down. That lightens the load on joints and muscles, making the senior years much easier with regards to mobility.

Does grocery shopping leave you out of breath? A regular strength workout will improve endurance and stamina and life will definitely get easier. The added energy makes for a good night's sleep after an active day. Insomnia will also be something of the past (Mayo Clinic, 2018).

Strength Training and Diseases

Several chronic and acute conditions can improve or be prevented through regular resistance training.

- **Heart Disease**

Strength training has been shown to help in lowering blood pressure, and reducing the load on the heart. The risk of cardiac arrest decreases when the heart is not under so much strain. That contributes to peace of mind which lowers stress levels, making your heart's environment even stronger (Mayo Clinic, 2018).

- **Diabetes**

Regular exercise helps to regulate insulin that keeps blood sugar levels under control. Researchers have found that physical activity increases the effectiveness of the protein APPL1, which plays an integral role in the absorption of glucose (Upham, 2018).

- **Arthritis**

Resistance exercise can alleviate joint stiffness and lessen pain, because the surrounding muscles are getting stronger. That leads to a vastly improved quality of life for those with arthritis (Mayo Clinic, 2018).

- **Asthma**

The severity and frequency of asthma attacks can be positively influenced by regular exercise, because lung function and capacity improve with resistance training (Mayo Clinic, 2018).

- **Back Pain**

Much of the back pain older people suffer is due to weakness of the supporting muscles. Targeted resistance exercises strengthen them while improved flexibility minimizes the strain put on the spine during movement.

- **Cancer Recovery**

One of the most debilitating symptoms cancer survivors have to contend with is overwhelming fatigue and weakness. The gentle and adaptable nature of a resistance band workout helps with overall recovery to increase stamina according to the individual's physical condition.

- **Dementia**

Regular physical activity and the accompanying higher oxygen content in the blood can improve cognitive function in individuals with dementia (Mayo Clinic, 2018).

Increasing Anaerobic Endurance

Anaerobic exercises like resistance training use muscle energy without oxygen, as opposed to aerobic exercises that need a constant supply of oxygen (Kelly, 2015).

Examples of aerobic exercises are fast-paced activities like jogging or swimming. Anaerobic activities use slower, shorter bursts to access the glucose in muscles without using oxygen. This stimulates bone growth, increasing density, and keeping osteoporosis at bay. It also improves overall bodily strength and endurance, making daily life that much easier to negotiate. It also increases the body's ability to handle lactic acid, which in turn increases your stamina for workouts (Kelly, 2015).

The Cardiovascular and Pulmonary Systems

Our hearts and lungs are among the first organs to really show signs of wear and tear in later years. Strength training can help you turn the clock back somewhat, even when battling a pulmonary infection or heart condition.

As joints and muscles get weaker with age, it becomes harder to move the body. That makes the heart and lungs work much harder to do the same things as before. A stronger body equals fewer aches and pains and more energy to enjoy life.

The lungs do not have to work so hard, because resistance training improves blood circulation and the available oxygen is utilized better.

As the circulatory system improves, metabolism speeds up and weight loss is kickstarted.

A Solution for the Whole Body

Resistance training offers a broad spectrum improvement package. Let's recap quickly.

- Muscles grow and become stronger, while joints are better protected and gain flexibility.
- Balance improves because muscles are stronger and joints move more easily.
- Pain is reduced because the body is stimulated into using its own healing mechanisms. A stronger frame that moves with less friction also limits everyday aches. Arthritis and lower back pain sufferers especially benefit from this.
- The heart, lungs, and circulatory system become more efficient.
- Bone density increases because bones are stimulated to grow. Studies have shown physical exercise

activates cells called osteoblasts. This chemical signal encourages deposits of calcium and other minerals necessary for bone growth (Weingart & Kravitz, 2020).

An "Anti-Aging Formula"

A study at the University of Birmingham (2018) found that a group of older lifelong amateur athletes had not undergone as much muscle and bone loss as people of a similar age who never exercised. Their cholesterol levels were also lower than expected, and their immune systems were stronger than the control group. The men had essentially avoided most of male menopause with their testosterone levels measuring significantly higher than their inactive counterparts in age.

Studies like these disproved the assumption that age makes us frail and that it is unavoidable. It is never too late to start a workout program and reap benefits for years to come.

Factors Affecting Success

Your strength workout success can be outlined by a few things. All of these issues are within your control and you can decide whether they will stand in your way or not.

Nutrition

Your diet will greatly affect your results, whether your main goal is weight management, fitness, or both. A balanced intake of food will supply your body with all the calories and nutrients needed for everyday activities with a workout thrown in. It is not only the type of meal that is important though, but also the time of day when it is eaten (Kilroy, 2014).

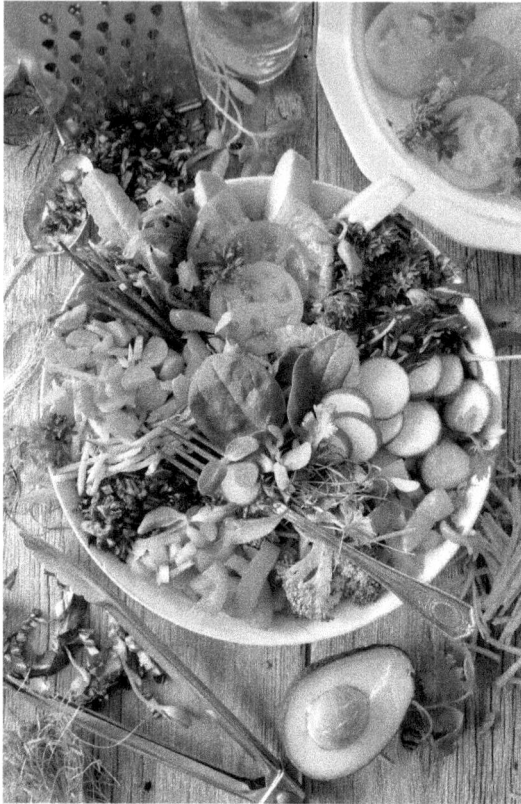

- **Breakfast**

Breakfast really is important, because it is the first meal after many hours without any nutrient absorption. Blood sugar levels are low and have to be restored to normal to supply fuel to your brain and body.

Protein plays an important role in this process. Simple and refined carbohydrates like a bagel on its own just won't cut it for long enough to get you through a workout without feeling lethargic and dizzy.

Instead, go for more complex carbohydrates with protein added like a slice of wholewheat toast with an egg or cheese. Avoid sugary cereals which can cause a blood sugar spike with a crash afterward, leaving you tired and feeling down. Rather go for oatmeal or whole-grain cereals with protein in the form of milk, yogurt or nuts added (Kilroy, 2014).

Carbohydrates supply more than half of our daily energy needs, despite the bed rap it has thanks to low carb diets. It should be complex carbs, however, which take longer to digest and keep us feeling full for longer. That is especially helpful in weight loss.

Examples of complex carbs are whole grain products, unprocessed foods, vegetables, fruits, and beans.

- **Snacks**

Your body needs food every two to four hours to keep blood sugar levels in the optimal range to supply energy for all activities, mental and physical.

Add a healthy snack to your diet mid-morning and mid afternoon, especially before exercising. The ideal snack contains protein and vegetables or fruit in small portions (Level et al., 2017). It could be for example a small piece of cheese and an apple, or a whole grain snack cracker with a slice of cold chicken or turkey on top.

A small amount of healthy unsaturated fat is also recommended. Go for a drop of olive oil on your toast and leave the butter (Kilroy, 2014).

- **Main Meal**

Your main meal of the day can contain bigger portions of protein and carbohydrates than the other two meals, in addition to a healthy portion of vegetables. It should preferably not be eaten just before going to bed, as the energy used by your digestive system to convert the food could interfere with sleeping. That will rob you of a good night's rest and leave your body with nutrients that can't be used as they should, ending up being stored as fat.

If possible, the biggest meal of the day should be consumed in the afternoon before 15:00 for the best weight loss and fitness results (Kilroy, 2014).

- **Pre-Workout Snacks**

Enjoying a snack containing balanced amounts of protein and carbohydrates just before starting your workout can ensure sustained energy throughout. That will avoid any sudden drops in blood pressure and sugar levels and provide the optimal physical environment to set you up for success.

Good candidates on this snack list are bananas, berries, grapes, oranges, nuts, and nut butters.

Protein is not called the building blocks of life for nothing. Protein molecules are broken down by the body into smaller molecules called amino acids (HEB, 2020). Amino acids are indispensable for muscle and tissue growth and repair.

How to Avoid the Weight Loss Stall

We all know losing weight depends on taking in less calories than before, so that our bodies can start using the stored fat reserves instead of just using the new calories and storing even more.

Sometimes even a tight hold on the number of calories eaten with regular workouts doesn't have the desired result. Weight loss just plateaus and nothing seems to get it going again.

- An important factor in this equation is the amount of stress you are under. Stress causes the secretion of the hormone cortisol from the adrenal glands (Kamau, 2020). Cortisol changes the way the body uses nutrients and can cause storage of energy as fat, instead of converting it into energy.
- Not getting enough sleep also changes your metabolic rate, which is the rate at which sugars are converted to energy (Kamau, 2020). Getting less uninterrupted sleep than what your body requires (on average about seven hours per night for adults) causes stress, which brings us back to the stress hormone cortisol. Most muscle growth also takes place during sleep, as well as repair to tissues. Strength training keeps on giving long after you finished your workout, working to build your new body while you rest.
- Water weight can be a contributing factor for seniors. Some medications cause water retention, as can eating too much salt and carbohydrates (Kamau, 2020).

- Once you start building muscle mass and bone density, your weight might also seem to stand still or even go up slightly. Don't be discouraged by this, you are winning the battle!

Body Composition

Your body consists of fat mass and fat-free mass. This is referred to as body composition (Tinsley, 2017).

Weight loss is affected by the changes in these two categories. If they change by the same amount at the same time, it stands to reason that no change in body weight will be detectable. For your resistance workout to be successful, you want the fat mass to decrease and the fat-free mass to increase. That is the formula for becoming the fitter, healthier and stronger you.

With the advice in this book you definitely are on the right road to achieving just that. It is within your reach to live a physically fulfilling and healthy life in your senior years. That will make it possible to stay independent for far longer and live life on your terms.

Chapter 5: Types of Resistance Bands and Specifications

There are many variations of resistance bands available, and they can be confusing to a first time user.

Each type has its own advantages and disadvantages, and experience will teach you which ones, or which combinations will suit your needs. If you look after them well, clean them regularly, and keep plastic and latex away from UV light when possible, you should get a long life of happy exercising from them.

For general purposes, a set of loops and a set of tubes with all the different resistant levels will be a good starting point to attain general fitness. As you progress through your workout routines, you will need to increase resistance to keep your muscles developing, and it is easier when you have the necessary equipment at hand without having to go to the store first.

If your aim with the workouts is to rehabilitate after an injury, therapy bands are probably a good starting point. They are gentle on weak muscles and long enough to be adequate for various exercise types.

The figure 8-band is versatile, and if you want to try with only one specialty band first on top of the basics, this is a dependent go-to for a wide variety of movements.

Attachments such as door anchors and ankle straps are nice to have but not essential in the beginning.

Do not worry; this chapter will provide a solid understanding of each type so you can make smart purchases and build your home gym to your advantage.

Loop Resistance Bands

Loop bands are exactly that - a continuous loop that is lightweight and versatile to use (Starwood Sports, n.d.). They are essentially big rubber bands. This type of band is popular to target and activate smaller groups of muscles that are sometimes overshadowed by their bigger neighbors and kept from getting a good workout.

Loop bands can also be added to others to change an exercise slightly or increase resistance. Exercises with loop bands can "wake up" muscles that have become lazy or strengthen stabilizing muscles to make movement safer.

This type of band comes in different colors, each with a different resistance level, although they are not available in ultra-heavy. Some core and upper body exercises are, therefore, not advisable with only loop bands (Simple Fitness Solutions, n.d.).

The same exercise can be done with all the different colors, increasing the intensity of the workout with every step up. They are also known as power bands.

They are available in different materials, from latex to rubber to material.

O-Shaped Expanders

Though these bands look like loops, they are generally shorter. They are good for lower body exercises. One disadvantage is that they tend to roll up around the ankles because they are fairly narrow, making them ineffective, and sometimes the skin gets pinched in the process (Simple Fitness Solutions, n.d.).

Tube Resistance Bands

The biggest difference between loops and tubes is that tubes are open-ended like skipping ropes, with handles. They can be made from thermoplastic or extruded rubber, or latex.

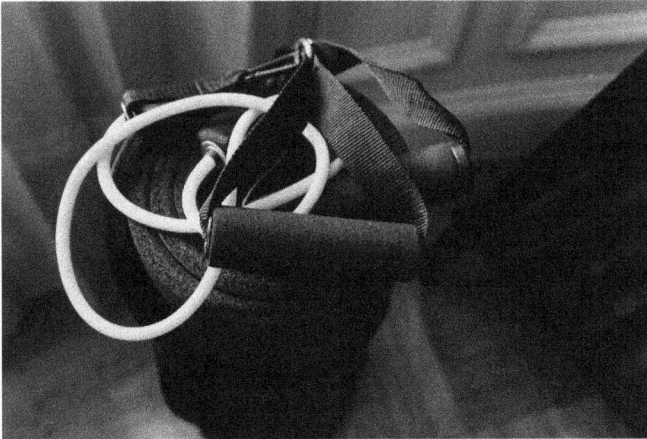

A tube with padded handles

Some have detachable handles while the handles of others are fixed. Handles can be padded or just plain hard plastic.

Some are also manufactured with clips at the ends to hook a variety of accessories for different exercises.

They are often longer than flat bands at about four feet, and the excess length can make them difficult to use when doing exercises like chest presses. In movements where only one handle is used, the other one can also get in the way.

Tubes are also not recommended for leg exercises on isolated muscles, because longer flat bands or pull-up bands provide more room for movement. Multi-joint exercises do not present the same problem.

Tubing with handles makes exercises where two sides must be worked at the same time more simple. When no door anchor is available, a handle makes a good substitute (Simple Fitness Solutions, n.d.).

Thermoplastic Rubber

This material is often used because it is a cheaper option. Thermoplastic rubber (TPR) is a man-made product with characteristics of both rubber and plastic, which makes it fairly strong. The manufacturing process is cheaper than the extraction of natural rubber, so it is used quite extensively.

It can be recycled, unlike natural rubber, because its block-like structure allows for recrystallization many times over (*What is Thermoplastic Rubber? (TPR)*, 2017).

Extruded Rubber

Extruded or natural rubber comes from rubber trees. The product is described as extruded because it is not molded into its final form like TPR. The soft and pliable rubber compound is fed into a die through an extruder, increasing pressure and temperature along the way to force the rubber through the openings in the die. The finished product is soft and has to be hardened in a process called vulcanization before it can be used (Timco Rubber, n.d.).

The main difference with TPR is in the distance a natural rubber band can stretch before it breaks. TPR can only stretch four or five times its length, while extruded rubber can be stretched up to six times its length. Natural rubber is also less susceptible to light degradation from UV rays (Garage Gym Reviews, n.d.).

Latex

Natural latex comes from the rubber tree in the form of a thick milky liquid. It is harvested by cutting strips of bark from the tree and allowing the liquid to drip into a container placed below the tree.

The harvest is then sent to a processing plant where it undergoes various processes to remove the water and stabilize the product. The concentrated latex contains about 60 percent rubber. Raw materials are then added to it to achieve the desired characteristics for the product.

Natural latex molds itself completely around anything such as plastic tubing dipped into it. Resistance tubes are formed by this process. (Sheppard, 2014). Dipped latex tubing can be stretched up to nine times their length (Garage Gym Reviews, n.d.).

If you have a latex allergy there are fabric alternatives available. The fabric makes the bands a little less stretchy than rubber or latex bands, which makes them ideal for lower body workouts.

Mini Hip Circle Resistance Bands

These sturdy exercise buddies are designed to strengthen the lower body. They are used around the legs, just above the knees, while different movements are performed. They are especially helpful to strengthen the hips and glutes.

A simple example of an exercise where a mini hip circle band is used to great effect is to place the band around your legs just above the knees and place your feet far enough apart so that some tension is detectable in the band. Then start walking forward and feel the tightness in the muscles put to work (Gunsmith Fitness, n.d.). This type of exercise holds great advantages for an older person seeking to regain strength, mobility, and flexibility in the hips. It prevents injuries and also improves balance.

Mini hip circle bands can be purchased in either fabric or non-fabric versions.

RENRANRING Resistance Bands

RENRANRING is a brand that offers latex as well as non-latex options, making their therapy bands a good option for hospitals and other facilities with a no-latex policy.

Online marketplaces like Amazon (Amazon, 2020) and Desert cart (Desert cart, n.d.) offer a whole variety of their products. There are complete sets of tubes with a door anchor, detachable handles, ankle straps, and a carry bag. They also manufacture sets of three open-ended flat bands with or without latex.

Figure 8 Resistance Bands

Also called a figure 8 expander, it is a loop that is fastened together in the middle in a figure eight form with handles on each end. It can be used around the feet or ankles for lower body exercises, around the hands or arms for the upper body, or in a combination of one side around the foot and the other around an arm or in the hand.

They are typically shorter than loop bands and prevent the wear and tear that looping a straight band can cause. The handles make them easier on the hands and also protect the bands from the shoes when looped around a foot.

The construction makes it somewhat easier for a band to snap or pull out of the center fastener, so exercise one arm at a time instead of both simultaneously (Mulrooney, 2011).

Letsfit Resistance Power Loop Bands

Letsfit is a company that specializes in making fitness and health information and accessories available to anyone. They offer sets with power loop bands as well as tubing in all the different strengths. There is also a product specifically developed to prevent rolling up with use (Letsfit, n.d.).

Therapy Bands

Used extensively for physiotherapy and to assist with home rehabilitation after an injury, therapy bands offer mostly light resistance although they are available in different strengths. They are flat bands that are not looped, and the average length is four feet.

They have exceptional elasticity and can be stretched up to 300 percent their own length (Dearden, 2017). Therapy bands are good starting points for resistance training where there is an existing injury, a medical condition, or if the person is frail. They can, however, be difficult to hold on to because they have no handles and no capacity to attach handles (Simple Fitness Solutions, n.d.).

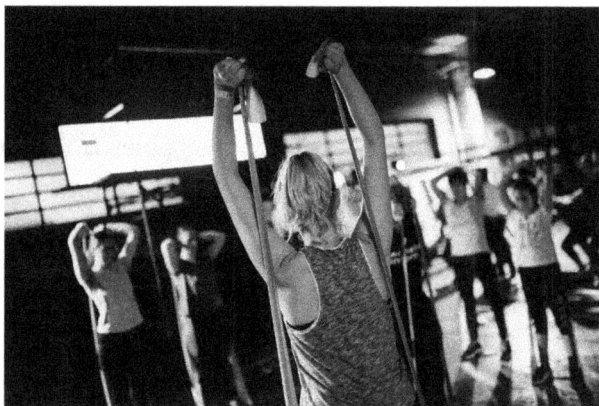

Theraband Resistance Therapy Bands

One of the well-known brands in this field is the company Theraband. They have been around for the last 40 years and pioneered the flat open-ended resistance band as we know it today (Theraband, n.d.). They include tubing in their range. Tubing is the only product that contains latex, while all bands are latex-free (Theraband, n.d.). They also offer a limited range of accessories, such as a wall anchor station for loop bands.

Whatafit Resistance Therapy Bands

The Chinese company Whatafit lists some of its bestseller products as their complete sets of resistance bands (Whatafit, n.d.). Some sets include accessories such as a door anchor, ankle straps, and detachable handles for tubing. They also offer sets of long pull-up bands.

Perfect Peach Resistance Therapy Bands

An online company that took the needs of women specifically to heart, is Perfect Peach Athletics. Their resistance bands sport peach, pink, and lilac color codes instead of the usual colors to denote the different strengths. They also pride themselves on products that are designed to be soft on a woman's skin while not compromising on durability (Perfect Peach Athletics, n.d.). The bands are also offered in a fabric version.

Tribe Resistance Bands

Tribe latex resistance bands are offered in sets as well as single tubes and bands with the usual accessories like a door anchor, detachable handles, and ankle straps (Tribe Fitness USA, n.d.).

Valeo Resistance Bands

The company Valeofit promises affordable prices for good quality with all their merchandise. Their range of bands in different lengths and tubes with accessories is available on Amazon and also offers other rehabilitation products like squeeze balls (Amazon Valeofit Store, 2020).

EDX Resistance Bands

EDX USA has a fairly extensive range of bands, tubing, and accessories available, which grew out of the personal experience of one of their founders. Everything from flat bands to 8-bands, padded detachable handles, and sets are offered (EDX USA, n.d.).

Lux Fitness Resistance Bands

The company Lux Fitness offers wide, elastic bands with non-slip inner layers. The non-slip elastic fabric makes them stronger than plastic or latex and minimizes the possibility of bad smells and skin irritation. Although the bands are marketed as hip, they can be utilized on other parts of the body, according to their website (Lux Fitness, n.d.). Their range also includes tubing and detachable handles.

Ziftex Resistance Bands

This company currently has a limited range of products, which includes a set of looped resistance bands (Ziftex, n.d.).

Physioworks Resistance Bands

Physioworks is an Australian company specializing in a wide range of physiotherapy products. They also have a line of exercise equipment, which includes power loop bands, figure 8 bands, loop bands, and stretch resistance bands as well as accessories like door anchors and detachable handles (Physioworks, n.d.).

8-Shape Resistance Bands

These bands, also called expanders, in the shape of a figure eight, provide a somewhat more challenging workout with some exercises. It is also sometimes known as an ultra toner. They can replace an ordinary looped band that is just twisted into a figure eight, making it easier to keep the shape firmly in place during the exercise because the form is fixed.

Let's look at a couple of easy exercises (Freytag, 2014):

- Put the band in the middle of your shoes with a loop on each foot. Sidestep three or four times to the right and back, then to the left and back. This engages the muscles in the thighs, buttocks, and hips.
- Wear the band in the same way as in the previous exercise, but squat down as low as you can while keeping resistance between your feet tight. Do five to eight repetitions.
- A variation on the exercise above is to stand with your heels together and your toes pointing outwards, before squatting.
- Hold the band in your hands, and pull the loops away from each other across your chest. Keep your back straight, and your shoulders relaxed and down.
- Engage your core muscles in the exercise above by lifting one foot off the ground while pulling the band open.
- Loop one ring around one foot and hold the other ring in your opposite hand. Push your foot away from you while pulling on the band with your arm. Keep your back straight, your shoulders relaxed, and your chin level.

Let your imagination invent more exercises for this versatile resistance band. Many everyday activities can be mimicked while wearing it. If you are traveling and have to keep your luggage as light as possible, an 8-shape band can replace some of the other bands and accessories.

BFR Bands

Simply put, blood flow restriction (BFR) training partially restricts blood flow to certain muscles during exercise to provoke muscle adaptation (BfR Professional, 2018). When used correctly, the restriction band should only obstruct the surface veins without affecting the deeper arteries at all.

According to BfR Professional (2018), the main advantage of this type of training is that the same results can be achieved with lighter workouts as with much heavier routines and weight lifting. They emphasize the need for proper warm-ups before starting occlusion training and to listen to your body and not overdo it because longer sets with shorter rest periods can be performed.

Superpump BFR bands

One of the brands available online through Amazon is Superpump (*Amazon.com : SUPERPUMP BFR BANDS | Simple + Effective Quick-Release Straps for Blood Flow Restriction Training and Kaatsu Style Workouts | Arms : Sports & Outdoors*, 2020). They offer comfort with a military-grade hook and loop closure for durability.

Resistance Band Rollers

A variation on traditional resistance tubes is adding a roller at each end with a pad on which to kneel or stand in the middle. This allows for a greater variety of exercises.

Foam Rollers

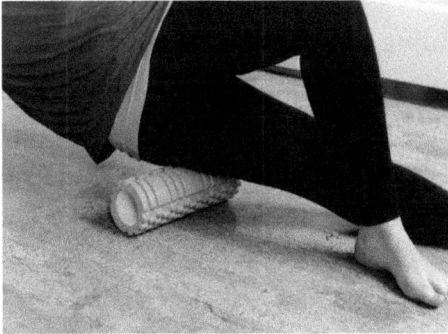

Foam rolling is another technique often used to release tension and increase range of motion. Used as a rehabilitation tool, it has also been added at the end of workouts as part of the cool-down (Victoria, 2016). The roller can be applied to all the points that trigger pain and the amount of pressure is determined by yourself.

According to Anna Victoria (2016), foam rolling or self-myofascial release can be especially beneficial for the lower body, abs, and back, and not much more than a five-minute routine is needed. It helps to increase blood flow and speeds up circulation, thereby preventing and breaking down scar tissue at the sites of injuries.

After a long day, rolling for a few minutes just before going to bed can ease built-up tension and pave the way for a restful night's sleep.

Many different brands are available online and in fitness stores, but if you can't purchase one, there are cheap and easy alternatives (*No Foam Roller? No Problem! Try These Alternatives! | ISSA*, n.d.).

- According to ISSA (n.d.), any ball like a tennis ball can be used as a substitute for a roller. If a tennis ball is too soft, a baseball will also do. The smaller surface of a ball works better when you lie down on the floor or press the ball against a wall. There are also dedicated massage balls available in different shapes, styles, and sizes.
- A kitchen rolling pin with something soft like dishcloths wrapped around it to soften the touch somewhat can also be used.
- A broomstick can target smaller areas and pinpoint scar tissue.
- Any hard bottle or a softer one filled with water will provide the same relief from tension and muscle aches. The harder the object is used, the more intense the pressure will be, and the deeper the massage will be.

Pull-Up Bands

Pull-up bands are the real heavyweights of the resistance band tribe. They have to be long but strong enough to hold an average person's weight and assist with pulling yourself up from the floor for certain exercises.

Grebest is one of the brands available online through Amazon (Amazon, n.d.). They offer lifetime durability in natural latex, with a return policy in case you are not satisfied with the product. The bands are also available in different resistance levels.

Long Bands

Some exercises like squats, pull-ups, and any movement requiring assistance will need a longer band to perform them comfortably. The shorter bands are also not suitable to anchor on a door, for instance.

If you are new to fitness or require a fair amount of assistance, a blue band offering a resistance of around 10 to 15 pounds. That provides a helping hand while still remaining challenging (Set for set, 2019).

They are also sometimes called assistance bands.

Kinetic Leg Resistance Straps

Sometimes foot injuries or certain foot conditions need the foot to remain upright and flat while stretching the Achilles tendon or calf muscle for the exercise to work properly without causing more damage. A resistance band with a strap that goes around the foot at one end is an effective way to ensure this.

It can also be worn while sleeping to keep on providing a gentle stretch to relieve pain caused by stress fractures in the heel and assist with correcting gait problems. It can be very useful when ankle flexibility is an issue (SoCal Health, n.d.).

Door Anchors

For some exercises to be effective, the bands need to be anchored around or under something. If you do not want to go to the trouble of fixing a permanent hook to a wall, there are cheap and easy ways to get around the problem.

A heavy piece of furniture can help you out, but you have to be sure it is really heavy. You do not want a piece of furniture to come flying at you.

A practical way to anchor your bands is by using a door anchor. It consists of a band with a loop at one end, into which a block is put. The band slides under the door with the block at the back of the door, catching there and making it possible to do exercises with heavy tension safely.

The band can also be inserted between the door and the jamb, with the anchor behind the door. This allows for variety in heights (Matt, n.d.).

In a pinch, you could fashion your own anchor out of an old T-shirt or belt just make sure the material is strong enough and that your knots will hold.

Ankle Straps

One of the useful accessories available for resistance bands is a sturdy wide ankle band with a clip attached. It is a safe and comfortable way to do leg exercises, minimizing strain on the ankles.

Handles

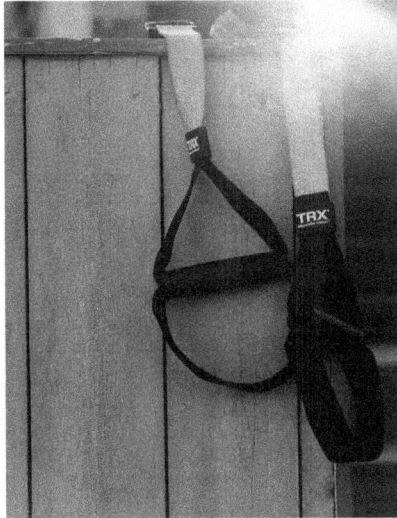

Handles are usually found on tubes rather than flat loop bands, although loop bands are occasionally fitted with handles too. The types of exercises usually done with loop bands make handles somewhat awkward to use though. Tubes are also rated for heavier resistance than bands, so handles make it easier to use the tube properly without discomfort (Harwood, 2018).

Handles can be made from hard plastic, or come in padded versions. Padding makes them softer on the hands. Padded handles consist of a nylon webbing pouch with a plastic handle with foam padding around it inside.

If the handle is equipped with a hook to attach it to different tubes, the hooks are manufactured from steel.

Chapter 6: Resistance Band Series Exercises

I bet you're itching to start applying everything you've learned by now, and you should have all the proper gear in place to do so. It's time to start moving!

Before getting into designing your own workouts or even following along with guided ones, we should pay some attention to all the different movements and their functions. One of the first concepts we need to look at is the different body parts that need to be trained and are grouped together for practical purposes.

The Main Body Parts

We can group exercises for the upper body, core, lower body, back, and abdomen.

Upper Body

The primary body parts and muscles in the upper body include the neck, shoulders, arms, chest, and upper back (Weight Loss Resources UK, n.d.).

Neck

We often don't give our necks a second thought until pain is present, but it is a vital part of our bodies. Weak neck muscles have an important impact on well-being in seniors.

The neck is a conduit between the brain and the spinal cord and there is not much padding in the form of muscles to protect this important passage. Fatigued and weak neck muscles can affect nerve impulses and hamper functioning and movement. Compromised neck muscles can even affect the quality of breathing (Kelso, n.d.).

Exercising and stretching the neck muscles are super easy and quick, and you reap immediate benefits in feeling better.

- Chin on chest: Bend your head forwards and try to push your chin into your chest. Hold for a couple of seconds and relax. For added oomph, fasten one end of your resistance band around your forehead and hook the other end around an anchor before pulling forward against it.
- Look up towards the ceiling, tilting your head back as far as is comfortable for you to do. With the resistance band positioned as in the previous exercise, you can also pull against the band to make the exercise a bit more challenging.
- Move your head from one shoulder to the other, flexing your neck as far as possible without pain. Pull against the resistance band if it doesn't hurt you to do so.
- Look to the right and the left as if you are about to cross a busy street. Turn your head as far as possible to each side and use your resistance band here (Kelso, n.d.).

Shoulders

The main muscles in the shoulders are the deltoids, which are at the top, and the rotator cuffs at the bottom (Weight Loss Resources UK, n.d.).

As we age, we often lose strength and toning in the upper body quickly because we don't lift and push things as often anymore while our legs still carry our body weight for a workout.

- Shoulder press for the deltoids: Use a long band or tube and stand in the center of it. Raise your hands to shoulder height. With the band behind your arms, bend your elbows at 90 degrees with palms facing outwards. Straighten your arms towards the ceiling. If it is impossible to get your arms into a straight position, you can lighten the resistance (Dick's Pro Tips, 2019).
- External rotation for the rotator cuff: Attach your resistance band to an anchor at belly button height. Stand perpendicular to the band and take it in your outside hand. Pull the band away from the anchor while keeping your elbow against your body. You can pinch a towel between your body and elbow to make sure your elbow doesn't move away (Set for Set, 2017).
- Wall crawl: Attach a short looped band around your wrists and lean your forearms against a wall. Keeping your shoulder blades as low as possible, crawl your forearms up the wall until the band is at eye level (Set for Set, 2017).
- Shrug: Stand with your arms by your sides. Pull your shoulders up as high as possible, squeezing your shoulder blades together at the top. For added resistance, you can fasten two bands to something near the floor and hold them taut before pulling your shoulders up.

- Front raise: Kneel with a resistance band looped under one knee. Pull the band straight up to shoulder height with one hand. Lower the arm slowly and repeat with the other arm (8fit Team, n.d.).
- Lateral raise: Do exactly the same as in the previous exercise, but pull the band out to the side, perpendicular to the body (8fit Team, n.d.).
- Seated row: Sit on the floor with your legs straight out in front of you. Loop the band around your feet and pull your hands back to your sides (8fit Team, n.d.).
- Lawnmower: This exercise imitates starting a lawnmower and is extremely easy to perform with resistance bands. Anchor the band in front of you or stand on it. Keep it fairly short and pull backward and up, as if trying to start a lawnmower with a pull cord. Alternate sides. It is also good for the back (Picincu, 2020).

Arms

An arm workout also benefits the shoulders, chest, and back. Only one band is needed for all the exercises.

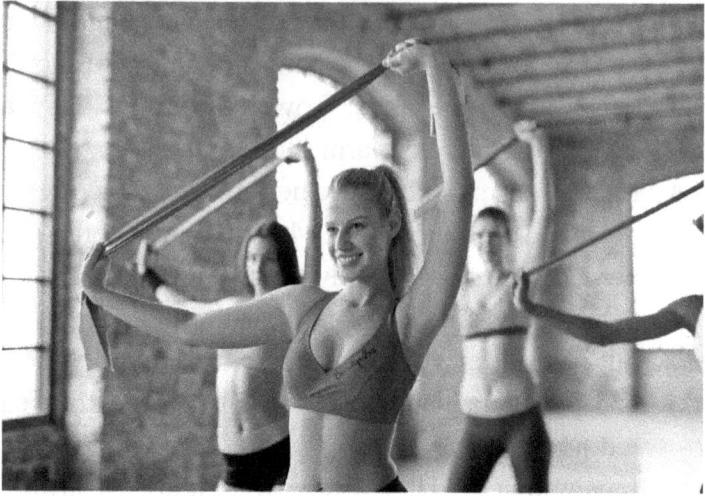

Try to do ten repetitions. The seventh and eighth should feel challenging, but you should still be able to finish the set. If you glide through all of the repetitions without feeling tired, it is time to move up to a band with more resistance (Eisinger, 2019).

- Seated biceps curl: Sit on a chair with one end of the band under your left foot. Take the other end in your right hand and rest your right elbow on your thigh. The band should be taut. Keep your back straight and pull your right hand up towards your right shoulder with the palm facing upwards. The bicep muscle is located on the front of the upper arm, and you should feel it working to pull the band up (Eisinger, 2019).
- Reverse curl: Do exactly the same as in the previous exercise, but turn your palm to face down (Eisinger, 2019).
- Flexion: Sit down and anchor the resistance band in front of you, level with your knees. Place your hands on your knees, hold one end of the band in each hand

with your palms facing upwards. Flex your wrists upward, pulling the band and feeling the muscles in both the wrist and the forearm contracting (Eisinger, 2019).

- Archery pull: This exercise imitates pulling a bow to shoot an arrow and reaches muscles that are not used in many everyday activities. Hold a looped band out in front of you perpendicular to your body. Pull the front end away from you as if drawing a bowstring. Hold the position for a few seconds and relax (Barber, 2018).

- Tricep extension: The triceps are at the back of the arms. Stand with one foot slightly in front of the other and with the center of the band under the back foot. Hold the ends of the bands in your hands and pull them up straight above your head. Slowly lower the ends behind your head until your elbows are bent 90 degrees. Move your arms up again slowly (Eisinger, 2019).

- Chair triceps dip: Anchor a band at a point high against a door or wall. Sit on a chair in front of the band and take the ends of the band in your hands. Gently pull down as far as possible (Eisinger, 2019).

- Overhead triceps extension: Stand on the center of the resistance band and pull the ends up until your hands are over your shoulders with your elbows pointing forward. Extend your arms in a straight line and bring them down again. Repeat five to eight times (Biswas, 2018).

Chest

The main muscles in the chest are the pectorals. They connect the front of the chest with the bones in your shoulder and upper arm.

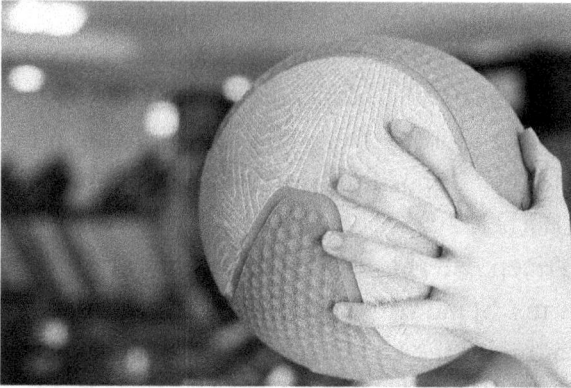

Small fitness balls can add resistance in chest exercises

- Chest press: Wrap a band around your body, chest height. Push the band out in front of you until your arms are straight. Hold for a few seconds and relax (Rubberbanditz, 2019).
- Incline press: Do exactly the same as in the previous exercise, but push your arms up at an angle instead of straight out in front of you (Rubberbanditz, 2019).
- Chest fly: Loop a resistance band around your body and stretch your arms out in front of you. Keeping tension tight in the band, pull your arms back as far as possible. Hold for a few seconds and relax (Rubberbanditz, 2019).
- Reverse chest fly: Do the same exercise as above, but start with your arms at the back and bring them forward slowly (Rubberbanditz, 2019).

- Pull down: Anchor the band high enough so that it is pulled taut when you kneel holding the ends above your head. Bring your arms down to shoulder height, hold the position for a few seconds, and gently let your arms go up again (*Resistance Band Lat Pulldown*, n.d.).

Lower Body

The lower body includes the knees, which are a problem for many older people, as well as the pelvis. Weak pelvic floor muscles can cause bladder and bowel problems for women especially and are often neglected in exercise routines.

While the knees have tendons and not muscles, weak knees affect the strength of the legs and hips (Young, 2020). Women are quite susceptible to knee problems in later years, because of their wider hips. Wearing high heels in youth can come back to haunt you later because this constant elevated foot position tends to shift weight to the knees.

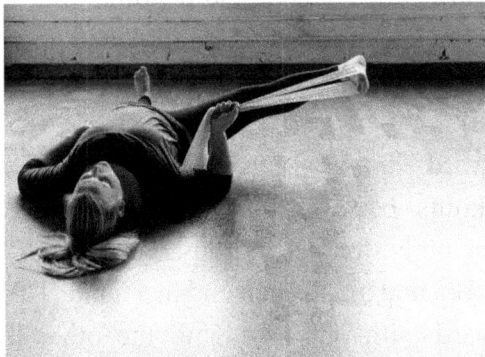

- The gas pedal exercise: This exercise was discussed in Chapter Three as part of the warm-up routine.

- Leg press: This exercise is best done in a seated position to keep the upper body and torso still and make balancing easy. Wrap the band around your feet and hold the ends just above thigh height. Push your legs straight out in front of you and bring them back again to the starting position. The exercise can also be done laying down if preferred (Nunez, 2018).
- Squats: Loop a resistance band around your shins and stand with your feet wide enough that some resistance from the band can be felt. Keeping your back straight, squat down with hips extended to the back while holding the distance between your feet. Hold your arms out in front of you or clasp your hands for balance. Come back up slowly in a controlled movement. When your thigh muscles are strong enough, you can widen the distance between your feet to do a sumo squat (Nunez, 2018).
- Squat shuffle: Place the resistance band just above your knees. Slowly go down into a squat stance, pushing your hips out and bending your knees. Keep your back straight, your feet flat, and your toes in line with your hips. Shuffle to one side and back (Nunez, 2018).
- Forward lunge: Lunges are an old favorite in workouts because they engage almost the entire lower body, as well as the core. Loop a band under one foot and grasp each end in a hand. Take a big step forward with one foot until the other knee almost touches the ground. Keep tension in the band all the time. Push yourself back up again to the starting position (Rubberbanditz, 2019).

- Sidestep: Loop a resistance band around your ankles while your feet are shoulder-width apart. Take a large step to one side, well outside your shoulders. Pause there for a moment, then step with the other foot in the same direction. Keep stepping for three or four paces before returning to the starting point (Rubberbanditz, 2019).
- Leg curls: This exercise concentrates on the hamstrings. Sit on a chair and anchor your band in front of you. Loop the other end around one ankle. Keep your feet together and pull your legs back as far as they can go before returning to the starting position (Nunez, 2018).
- Leg abduction: Lie on your back with a band looped around your feet and the ends in your hands. Keep your elbows on the ground beside you. Open your legs wider than your hips and bring your feet back again to the starting position (Spark People, n.d.).
- Hip extension: Loop the band around your ankles. Extend one leg behind you as far as possible, keeping it straight. Return to the starting position slowly and in a controlled manner (Nunez, 2018).

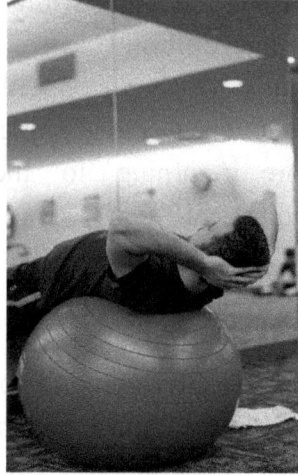

Effective core training strengthens much more than just your six-pack or rectus abdominis. It engages all the muscles that wrap around the abdominal area, as well as the pelvis, hips, back, and glutes (Atemi Sports, 2019).

- Chair sit-up: Sit on a chair with a band looped around your ankles. Keep your lower back as straight as possible, and bend forward to move your chest towards your thighs. Keep your feet flat on the ground and keep the tension in the band constant. Come back up slowly and repeat five to eight times (Atemi Sports, 2019).
- Reverse wood chop: Anchor the band and hold the other end with both hands. Bend your knees slightly and pull the band across your body and up. Return to the starting position, keeping full control of the movement (Train With Me Fitness Inc, n.d.).
- Side bend: Grasp the band at the ends and extend your arms above your head while keeping the band

stretched tight. Bend to one side and keep the tension in the band. Keep the position for a few seconds before bending to the other side. Keep your body straight all the time (Fit Carrots, n.d.).

- Pelvic lift: This exercise is performed while lying on the back with a resistance band looped around the knees. Lift your hips into a bridge position and gently push your knees out against the resistance of the band. Repeat the movement with toes pointing inward and outward (Watkins, 2014).
- Push-ups: Loop a resistance band around your upper body, under your arms. Lie down on your stomach and push your upper body up on your arms. You can also bend your knees instead of keeping your legs straight to make the exercise somewhat easier (Fit Carrots, n.d.).

The Back

Many back pain sufferers will find relief when their back muscles and other supporting muscles are strengthened enough to carry their weight with ease. Resistance band training is an excellent and safe way to achieve this.

- Lat pull-down: Loop a resistance band around your wrists and extend your arms above your head. Push your hands away from each other while lowering the band behind your shoulders. Return to the starting position (Cordeau, n.d.).
- Pull-apart: Hold the ends of a resistance band with your arms stretched out in front of you, and the band pulled tight. Pull your hands away from each other

while keeping your back absolutely straight. Return to the starting position (Cordeau, n.d.).

- Back fly lying: Stand with both feet on a band and tilt your body forwards. Extend your arms in front of your knees with palms facing each other. Pull your arms backward and out behind your body as far as possible. Keep the position for a few seconds before returning to the starting position (Patricie K, n.d.).
- Bent over rows: Place your feet on the band, hip-width apart. Bend forward at the waist and grasp the handles. Pull them up in a rowing motion with palms facing the body. Keep the back straight and lift the elbows towards the ceiling (Spark People, n.d.).
- Deadlift: Stand on the band and hold the ends with your palms facing backward. Push your hips down until you feel your hamstrings stretch. Keep your torso and back straight while pushing upright again slowly (Rubberbanditz, 2019).

The Abdominal Area

Muscles in the abdominal area influence breathing, posture, stability, and balance. When they are strong, everyday activities like bending down to tie your shoe or swinging a golf club become much easier.

Strong abdominal muscles can alleviate lower back pain and assist in maintaining the correct weight (EFM Healthclubs, 2018).

- Standing knee raising: Stand with your feet slightly wider than shoulder-width and place a resistance band around the middle of your feet. Lift one leg to your chest and try to touch your knee to your elbow without rounding your shoulders. Alternate legs (Mateo, 2017).

- Banana rolls: The trick with this exercise is never to let your hands and feet touch the floor. Lie on your front with hands and feet lifted off the floor. Position a resistance band around your ankles. Roll over onto your back, keeping the tension in the band. Roll back to your stomach while still keeping hands and feet clear of the floor (Mateo, 2017).
- Bicycle crunches: Loop a resistance band around the middle of your feet. Sit on the floor with bent knees and heels touching the floor. Lean back until you can feel your abdominal muscles working. Hook your fingertips behind your ears and twist your body to touch your right elbow to your left knee while straightening your right leg. Do the same with the other arm and leg to complete one repetition. Repeat five to eight times (Mateo, 2017).
- Side plank: This exercise could be fairly difficult for beginners, and you should listen to your body when attempting it. Pain anywhere means your muscles are not ready yet. Lie down on your side with one foot stacked on top of the other and a resistance band around your ankles. Push yourself up on the bottom arm with the heel of the bottom foot touching the floor. Lift the top leg up stretching the band, and try to hold the position for 30 seconds before relaxing and doing the same on the other side (Mateo, 2017).
- Plank hold: Another variation on the plank exercise is to loop a resistance band around your waist. Kneel on the floor with your palms down, and thumbs

hooked into the band. Support your body on one knee and push the opposite leg out straight to the back. Straighten the other leg as well and hold the position for a few seconds (Biswas, 2018).

- Spiderman push-up: This is another exercise that can be quite difficult in the beginning. Start in a push-up position with a resistance band around the middle of your feet. As you go down towards the floor, pull your right knee up towards your elbow. Alternate legs (Mateo, 2017).

- Sit-ups: Anchor the resistance band in front of you and lie down on the floor with the ends of the band in your hands. Bend your knees slightly and keep your feet flat on the floor. Pull yourself upright into a sitting position with the aid of the band and keep your back straight and your shoulders relaxed and down (Mateo, 2017).

Golfing Exercises

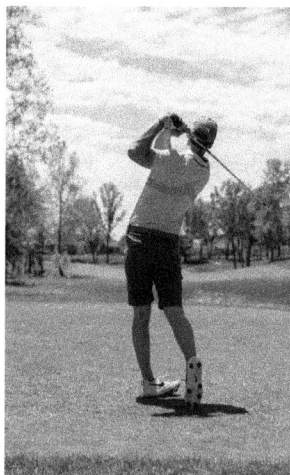

Although a golf club is not part of the body, ardent golfers in their senior years with enough leisure time to pursue this pastime might argue.

Resistance band training is especially beneficial to golfers to create consistency in their game or make more powerful swings. Even professional golfers have discovered the benefits of resistance bands in recent years, and trainers never leave home without them (Herman, 2017).

Targeted Warm-Ups

With resistance bands, you can target and tailor your warm-up routine to focus on any body part or muscle that is nursing an injury or is not as strong as you would like it to be.

The buzz word is prehabilitation, which is a shortened form of preventative rehabilitation. Exercises in this category not only warm up the targeted muscles and joints but also strengthen them at the same time to prevent injury further down the line. Shoulder rotator cuffs are an excellent example of the type of body part where golfers can use prehab to great advantage (Herman, 2017).

If you have to start a game while still sore from the previous day's activities, resistance band warm-ups at light resistance will help you ease into movement gradually and prevent injury.

Joint Stability

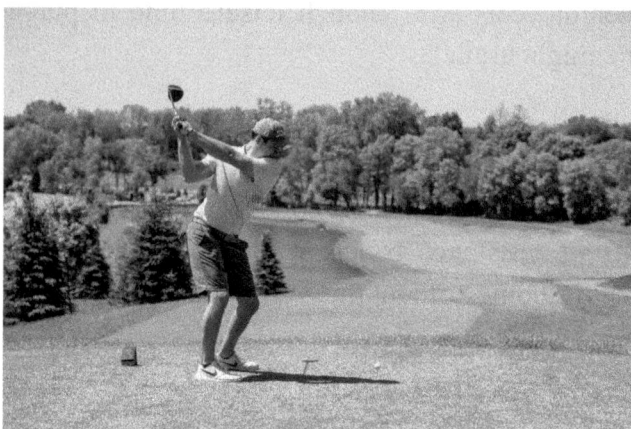

Stability and flexibility go hand in hand and become more and more important in later years. Golfers undergo a particular type of wear and tear to their joints due to repetitive movements, and loop bands can isolate the small groups of muscle around joints, to stabilize them (Herman, 2017).

The elasticity of the bands also supports a full range of motion to increase and maintain mobility in ways that weights and other types of exercises just cannot do.

The All-Important Swing

What is a golfer without his swing, you might ask? Whether you just want to improve or if there is an issue with your technique, resistance bands are perfectly suited to mold motor patterns and movements.

Trainers often use a type of reverse technique when a specific technical issue has to be modified. If the negative movement is initiated with a resistance band, the golfer is forced to move in the opposite direction, thereby executing the correct movement. Through cell memory, the new and correct motor pattern is laid down in the brain, and a revised technique starts taking shape (Herman, 2017).

Being so portable and lightweight, the bands can be carried into any change room and used on-demand without assistance from anyone else.

Fitness

As with any sport, golf requires a manner of fitness that is suitable for the demands of the sport. There are distances to be walked between holes to get the full benefit of being outside in the fresh air. If you do not have the luxury of a caddy, the heavy golf bag must also be carried around.

Arms and shoulders getting tired halfway through the game might just cost you the bottle of vintage wine up for grabs as a prize for the winner.

Let's look at some exercises that are recommended for golfers.

- Golfer's wood chop: Anchor your band behind you at about the point from where you would swing your golf club to play. Take the other end in both hands and perform a diagonal downward movement as if you are swinging a club. Make sure you stand far enough from the anchor point to create a fair amount of resistance against the downward swing and try to do it faster every time for two repetitions before switching sides. Perform three sets. Focus on controlled movement, not the type of strength that will hit the ball into the next county (Bowden, 2015)

- To strengthen the 'pushing' part of your golf swing, do the same exercise as above but only use your trailing arm (Bowden, 2015).
- The 'pulling' part of the swing can be exercised by repeating the previous exercise, but this time using your lead arm (Bowden, 2015).
- To work on your follow-through, anchor the band low and take the other end with your swing hand. Extend your arm upwards in the follow-through movement while pulling against the resistance of the band (Bowden, 2015).
- The impact with which the ball is struck can be exercised by taking hold of the band with the back arm and pulling it forward and downward, extending the triceps to the impact position (Bowden, 2015).

If you do these golf-specific exercises before going onto the green, you will have a great warm-up and be ready to play the game at your best.

Adding Accessories

You can add accessories like balls and dumbbells to many of the exercises described above to create variety and possibly even make them effective in a shorter time, depending on your own strength and where you are in your fitness journey.

Balls

Fitness or balance balls are a good accessory to your workout to help with stability and core strength. Balance ball resistance kits are available that consist of two resistance bands that fit over the ball for a more challenging workout.

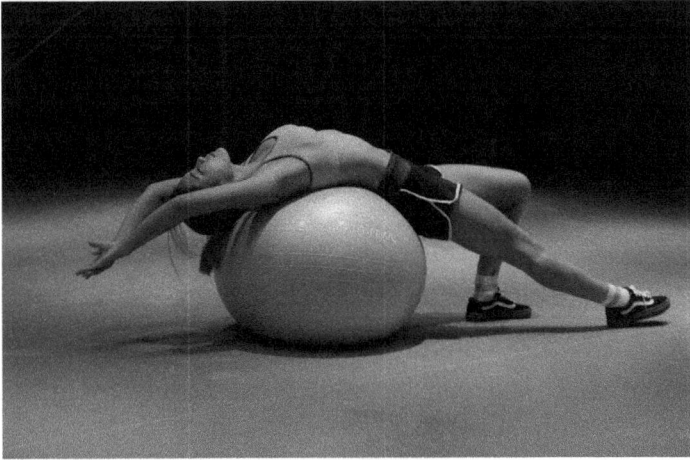

- Reclining fly exercise: Sit on the ball and hold on to the ends of the resistance band. Roll back until your back is on the ball and keep your feet flat on the ground. Straighten your arms, pulling on the bands. Hold the top position for a few seconds and relax (Skimble, n.d.).
- Upright fly: Do the same exercise as above, but stay upright. This version might be easier for anyone with back problems (Skimble, n.d.).
- Chest press: Sit down on the ball with the ends of the bands in your hands. Pull the bands up and over your chest. Lower your arms, but no lower than shoulder height (Waehner, 2019).
- Bench press: Do the same exercise as above while lying down on the ball (Waehner, 2019.

Dumbbells

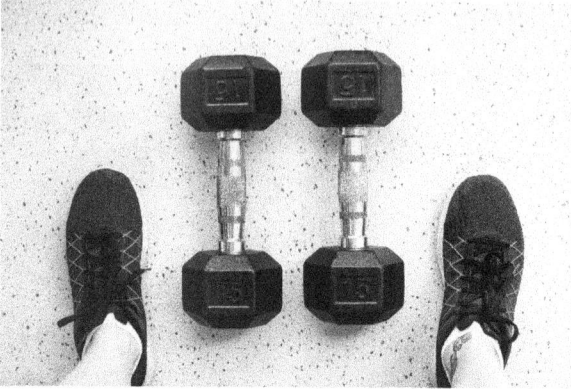

Widely used in strength training, these weights come in different sizes and can be used for a variety of different exercises. They consist of a handle with a weight on each side. The weights can be fixed or removable.

- Chest press: Loop a band around your back. Take the dumbbells one in each hand and press the band out with your hands on the inside of the band. Push the band and dumbbells up above your head and hold for a few seconds before relaxing (Skimble, n.d.).
- Chest fly: Lie on your back and loop a band around your wrists. Hold the dumbbells in your hands and rest your arms straight out to your sides at shoulder height. The band should be taut. Lift both arms straight up and bring them back down slowly (Skimble, n.d.).
- Lateral raises: Stand on the band and take a dumbbell and an end of the band in each hand. Raise your arms to the sides, up to shoulder height, and hold for a few seconds before relaxing (Bentley, 2016).
- Frontal raise: Do exactly the same exercise as above, but raise your arms in front of you instead of to the sides.

- Biceps curl: Stand in the middle of a band with a dumbbell in each hand and loop the ends of the band over the dumbbells. Pull the dumbbells up to shoulder height and hold for a few seconds before releasing (Brathwaite, 2018).

Chapter 7: Sample Core Workouts

In this chapter, you will find examples of core workouts that will help you achieve your desired results. It will help you see the pattern of a successful core workout and empower you to design your routines.

Remember, it is your life, make it interesting! Enjoy the road to greater health, fitness, and happiness. These examples are just starting points. Take a look at all the exercises in the book and play around with them until you have the perfect combination for you.

Core Workout 1

There are three exercises in this workout: The bicycle crunch, the mountain climber, and the hip thrust. Do them one after the other. Use 45 seconds per exercise with 15 seconds of rest in between. That brings you to a total workout time of nine minutes.

Bicycle Crunch

This vigorous exercise was discussed in Chapter Six under workouts for the abdominal area, but let's recap quickly.

It is best done sitting on the floor with bent knees and heels touching the floor. Position the resistance band around the middle of your feet and lean back until you can feel your abdominal muscles tugging and stretching. Keep them tight.

Hook your fingertips loosely behind your ears and twist your body to touch your right elbow to your left knee while straightening your right leg. Do the same with the other arm and leg to complete one repetition (Mateo, 2017).

Adapt your tempo to your fitness level and any physical constraints you might have. If you feel up for it, you can increase the intensity by holding a weight like a dumbbell or even just a can of tinned food in your hands while touching your elbows to your knees.

Mountain Climber

The traditional mountain climber exercise is performed quickly. Adding the resistance of a band makes it slower and far more intense and effective. It also adds benefits for the hips.

Get down on the floor in a push-up position, with a mini band around your ankles. Pull one knee up towards your chest as if you are climbing a rock. Return to the starting position and repeat with the other leg to complete one repetition (Gomez, 2017).

Hip Thrust

Hip thrusts specifically target all the gluteus muscles in particular. The exercise isolates them in a more effective way than more general hip movements can.

Lie on your back with the band looped over your thighs. Pin the ends of the band on the sides of your body with your hands. Keep your knees bent and your feet flat on the floor. Push your hips up against the band.

If you want to add weight, you can put a dumbbell under the band on your tummy (Fit Carrots, n.d.).

Core Workout 2

This workout has four exercises: The low-high chop, the side plank row, the high leg raise, and the high plank row. They are to be performed as supersets consisting of three sets each with 12 to 15 repetitions in each set. By the seventh repetition of each movement, it should start feeling challenging; otherwise, you will have to increase the repetitions.

The total workout time should be 10 to 15 minutes.

Low-High Chop

The wood chop was discussed in the previous chapter under core exercises. It can be done from either a high or low starting point. For the greatest effectiveness in core training, it is best to start it from below.

Anchor the band close to the floor. Bend down and take hold of the other end with both hands. With slightly bent knees, pull the band across your body and up as if you are raising an ax to chop wood. Return to the low starting position, keeping full control of the movement (Train With Me Fitness Inc, n.d.). Controlled movement and a full range of motion are very important in this exercise.

To add intensity, you can hold a dumbbell in your hands and lift that as well.

Side Plank Row

Lie down on the floor on your side and in the plank position. The band must be attached to a point close to the floor level. Hold the ends of the band in your top hand and raise yourself into a plank. Perform a rowing motion with the top arm (Men's Health, 2011).

High Leg Raise

Lie on your back with a mini band looped around your ankles and your heels on the floor. Lift one leg as high as possible against the band's resistance while keeping the other leg still and your shoulders firmly on the floor.

Do the same with the other leg to complete one repetition (Atemi Sports, 2019).

High Plank Row

The trusty plank exercise for core strength works on more than 20 muscles at the same time. It minimizes the chances for a back injury and does not hold the risks of hip stress, unlike sit-ups (Andersen, 2014).

It is advisable to master the basic plank before attempting to add the row.

Anchor a band low on the floor in front of you and get into plank position while holding the ends of the band. Bend your elbow and pull your arm slowly towards the ceiling, all the while working against the resistance of the band. The elbow should remain close to your side. Repeat with the other side to complete one repetition.

Use a dumbbell in the hand that is lifting to add intensity (Andersen, 2014).

Core Workout 3

As with the previous sample workout, the four exercises in this example should be performed as supersets consisting of three sets each, with 12 to 15 repetitions in each set. By the seventh repetition of each movement, it should start feeling challenging; otherwise, you will have to increase the repetitions.

The exercises are the bicycle crunch, the mountain climber, the torso rotation, and the side plank reach.

Bicycle Crunch

This exercise remains the same as explained in the first core sample workout.

Mountain Climber

This exercise also remains the same as explained in the first core sample workout.

Torso Rotation

The same exercise was discussed in chapter three as the twister exercise and done slowly like described there, it is an excellent warm-up movement.

It has its place in any core routine though, because once the muscles are warmed up, the exercise can be performed somewhat faster for a more thorough workout.

The muscles targeted are the abdominals that provide support to the whole abdominal area. Weakness in these muscles can have a significant impact on back health.

The obliques next to the abdominals are conditioned at the same time. They play a stabilizing role and are just as important for posture and overall health (Train With Me Fitness Inc, n.d.).

While the body rotation done with only a resistance band provides a good workout, holding a dumbbell while rotating will add intensity when your fitness level allows it.

The exercise can also be done in a seated position if preferred, and the dumbbell can be substituted for a medicine ball or any other fairly heavy object such as a bag of flour or cans of tinned food.

You should sit with your feet off the ground and rotate from hip to hip (Train With Me Fitness Inc, n.d.).

Side Plank Reach

Start in a side plank position. With your free hand, hold on to a resistance band that's anchored at a low point behind your back. Pull the band under your body while rotating your rib cage at the same time so that you end up looking down at the floor. It is the same motion as if starting a lawnmower.

Keep your core muscles tight the whole time to prevent your body from rotating too far, and have you ending up flat on the floor.

For added intensity, you can hold a dumbbell in the same hand as the rope (Train With Me Fitness Inc, n.d.).

Other Exercises to Mix and Match

Many of the exercises already discussed in earlier chapters can be swapped out for great core workouts.

Mini-band exercises to consider are the banded squat, mountain climber, bicycle crunch, clamshell, glute bridge, hip thrust, lateral walk, leg abduction, psoas march, and push-ups. Let's look at them!

- Clamshell: This is a great exercise not only for strengthening the hip and core muscles but also for easing tension in the lower back. Lie on your side with your legs stacked and your knees bent at a 45-degree angle. Loop a resistance band around your legs above the knees. Rest your head on your lower arm and steady yourself with your upper arm to help stabilize your hips. Pull your belly button in towards your spine. Raise your top leg as high as possible without moving your hips or lifting your shoulders off the floor. Hold for 10 to 15 seconds and return to the starting position.

- Psoas march: The psoas muscle is one of the hip flexors and influences balance and mobility greatly. To do the exercise, you should lie down on your back with your hips up in a vertical position, your knees bent, and your feet flexed so your toes point to the ceiling. Loop a resistance band around your feet. Take a deep breath and while exhaling, stretch one leg out in front of you and lower it to the lowest point where you can still control the movement. The other leg should remain still, as should your ribcage, shoulders, and pelvis. For added intensity, you could lie with your head close enough to a wall to press your palms against the wall behind your head, fingers pointing towards the floor (Callaway, 2018).

For some exercises, the assistance of a pull-up band is required. These are longer and stronger bands, but they make excellent aids when an extra helping hand is needed.

Here are a few to get you started:

- Band-assisted pistol squats: If you're feeling adventurous and strong, you can try this one-legged squat. Experts warn, however, that you have to be sure you have the strength to complete at least three sets of 15 regular squats before even attempting to do a pistol squat (Carpenter, 2020). Anchor your band high up in front of you and take hold of the ends with both hands. Lift one foot and go down in a squat on the other leg while holding on to the band. Keep your core muscles engaged and your back and ankles straight. In the beginning, you can place a low chair behind you and go down to the chair until you're strong enough to do it without any halfway stop.
- Band-assisted pull-ups: Pull-ups test the back and arms and the use of a resistance band can make the exercise considerably easier to perform. Anchor the band in front of you. The length should be such that your feet do not touch the ground if you stand on the band. Hold on to a bar or something similar above your head and pull your body up as far as possible. Ideally, you should be able to elevate your whole head and neck above the bar. Use smooth movements, no jerks. Don't lift your chin and strain

your neck, let your arms, shoulder, and back do the work. Lower yourself slowly again (Arana, 2019).

- Stationary band-resisted sprints: Bands can be used either as assistance or resistance. For this exercise, the resistance will be utilized. It is an excellent way to increase stamina and endurance and will also assist in burning calories if you want to manage your weight. Simply anchor your band behind you and loop the band around your waist. Then try as hard as you can to run forward, straining against the band. For added resistance, you can add a mini-band above your knees as well (Pridgett, 2019).

- Assisted hip hinge: This exercise focuses on the backside of the core muscles. It is also sometimes called the dowel rod hinge. The muscles targeted are essential for everyday activities where hips are bent, such as picking something up from the floor. The bending movement must come from the hips and not the waist. Place a band around your waist and anchor the band behind you. When you pull against the band, it will help you into a bent position. You have to engage your core muscles to come upright again while keeping your back straight. You must feel your hamstrings contracting during the movement. Do not let your knees go past your toes (The Prehab Guys, n.d.).

- Assisted skater squats: This exercise is not only good for the hips and legs but also promotes ankle stability. It is quite a vigorous movement. Loop a mini-band around above your knees. Then jump lightly from side to side, controlling your landing tightly and landing softly. Keep the tension in the band, and do not close the gap between your knees (Lugo, 2017).

You now have a solid foundation from which you can start a proper workout program, but also begin building and designing your own similar workouts according to your preferences, physical condition, and lifestyle.

Don't hesitate to begin mixing and matching these movements into fun and interesting groupings that will keep you excited when you think about your exercise program.

Chapter 8: Designing Your Own Programs

Now we have come to the really exciting and fun part of the book! You know enough of resistance training now to start putting together your own routines. This is where you get to mix and match any exercises that work for you.

I have a couple of suggestions to get you started, but you are the one in the driving seat from here on.

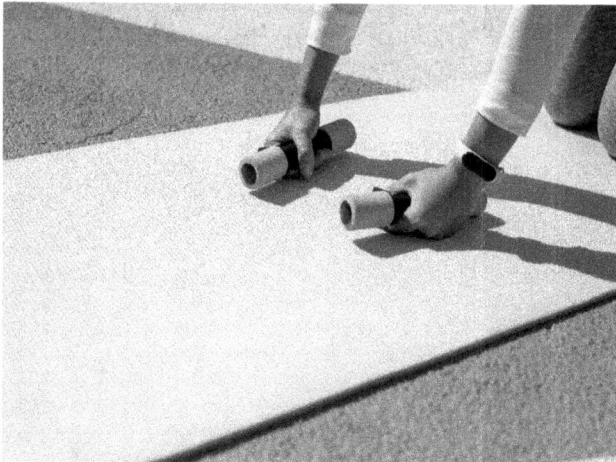

Two Workouts per Week Program

Day One

The exercises should be performed as supersets, consisting of three sets with 10 to 15 repetitions each. The workout should take about 40 minutes.

- Chest press: One version of this exercise was explained in chapter six, but there are other ways of doing it just as effectively. It can be done in a standing, sitting, or lying down position. Instead of pushing your arms out, you can move your body. Anchor the band near the floor and grab hold of the ends. Move your body forward into a lunge position and pull the bands with you until your arms are parallel to the floor at shoulder height. This is a forward and upward movement at the same time (Hoffman, 2020).

- Standing row: This exercise provides a thorough workout for the shoulders and upper back. Anchor the band at chest height and hold the ends so that your hands are slightly in from shoulder width. Stretch your arms out and pull the band towards your belly button while allowing your hands to move away from each other. Stop after reaching your body and return to the starting position. Concentrate on keeping your head and neck relaxed and allow your shoulder blades free movement (The Movement Fix, 2018).

- Glute bridge: The trusty and simple glute bridge in its basic form as discussed in an earlier chapter is a very versatile movement that can be performed in a variety of ways (Salyer, 2016). When the toes are pointed outward instead of facing forward, a different set of the glutes receive the workout. For more variations, the heels can be pressed down and the toes lifted, or the toes can be pressed down and the heels lifted. The movement can also be performed with only one foot on the floor and the other leg stretched straight up. Placing a weight on your abdomen during the exercise immediately ramps up the intensity (Salyer, 2016).

- Lateral walk: Also known as monster walks and banded shuffles, these mini-band side steps can prevent or alleviate knee pain when performed correctly. There are variations on the basic version discussed earlier in the book. If you use a large band rather than a mini-band and stand on it with the loop crossed in front of you, you engage your shoulders as well. You could also combine the walk with weights in the hands and another mini-band looped around the wrists (Maximum Training Solutions, 2016).
- Arnold press: This all-round multi-joint exercise has not cropped up before in our discussions. Stand or sit with a straight back and loop a mini-band around your wrists. You can either hold a weight in each hand or do the movement without additional weights. Start with your hands on your shoulders and lift your arms until they are straight while rotating your palms. When you get to the top of the movement, your palms should be facing each other. You can also do one arm at a time or alternate them (Arnold Press - How to Do It, n.d.).
- Banded squat: This exercise was discussed in Chapter Six.
- Mountain climber: This exercise was discussed in the third core workout in Chapter Seven.
- Side plank row: This exercise was discussed in Chapter Seven and does require some level of fitness before attempting.

Day Two

The exercises should be performed as supersets, consisting of three sets with 10 to 12 repetitions each. The workout should take about 40 minutes.

- Kneeling pull-down: This exercise was discussed in chapter six. It is worth noting that it can be done by either standing on one knee or both.
- Split squat: Place the middle part of one foot on a band and place the other foot a step behind. Pull the band up towards your shoulders with your elbows pointing towards the floor. Bend both knees to go down in a lunge position before coming upright again (Skimble, n.d.).
- Chest press: As done in day one's program.
- Single-leg deadlift: A variation on the explanation in chapter six is to do the deadlift with only one leg. Loop a resistance band around your ankles. Bend one knee slightly and extend the other leg behind you to help keep your balance. Hold for a few seconds and return to the starting position (Soto, 2018).
- Overhead press: This is an excellent way to tone and strengthen shoulders and arms. Stand on a resistance band with your feet shoulder-width apart. Hold the ends of the band and raise your hands to your shoulders and elbows out to the side. Then raise your arms straight up, working against the resistance of the band. Lower your arms again to shoulder height and repeat the exercise (Sworkit Wellness, n.d.).
- Hip thrust: A slight variation on the version that was discussed in the previous chapter is to sit on the floor with your shoulders and upper arms resting on

something like a bed or soft chair. Loop a band around your thighs and under your shoes. Thrust your hips upward so that your body pulls into a straight line, except for your knees that remain bent at a 90-degree angle. Keep your back straight, and imagine you squeeze a coin between your buttocks as you lift your hips. You could also kneel with the band anchored behind you and lean forward before thrusting your hips out, or stand bent at the waist while pulling the band forward between your legs and pushing yourself upright (BIQ Band Training, 2020).

- Bicycle crunch: This is a staple exercise that crops up in many workout routines. See the discussion in the previous chapter.

- High-low chop: Doing the movement this way round is exactly the opposite of the low-high chop that was discussed in the second sample core workout in the previous chapter.

Three Workouts per Week Program

Day One

The exercises should be performed as supersets, consisting of three sets with 10 to 12 repetitions each. Make sure the seventh repetition becomes challenging. The workout should take about 40 minutes.

- Quadruped kickback: The exercise is also known as quadruped hip extension or glute kickback. It is one of the easier movements for beginners or people without much physical strength. Kneel on the floor and place your hands under your shoulders. Keep your knees positioned under your hips. Lift your knee until your upper leg is parallel with the floor while keeping your knee still bent at a 90-degree angle. Then straighten your leg completely before reversing the process (Williams, 2020).

- Single-leg deadlift: The same as in the previous routine.
- Face pull: Contrary to what the name might suggest, this has nothing to do with your expression. It is basically a shoulder and back strengthening exercise which is done by pulling a band towards your face. Looped bands work best. Anchor it at head height and pull your elbows back, keeping them shoulder height. As your hands get closer to your face, you also pull them apart from each other. Then move back to the starting position in a controlled, smooth movement (Rusin, 2017).
- Push-ups: These need no introduction and have been discussed earlier in the book.
- Standing row: See earlier discussion in the section about day one of the previous programs.
- Banded squat: See the discussion on lower body exercises in chapter six.
- Hip raise: This is just another name for the hip thrust exercise that was discussed earlier.
- Bicycle crunch: See earlier discussions.

Day Two

The exercises should be performed as supersets, consisting of three sets with 10 to 12 repetitions each. Make sure the seventh repetition becomes challenging. The workout should take about 40 minutes.

- Skater squats: This exercise was discussed at the end of the previous chapter.
- Pull-through: When doing hip hinges, it is easy to fall into movement patterns that do not have the desired effect. The pull-through exercise that is done with a long band can prevent that. When done regularly, it will reinforce the correct way of movement for healthy and strong hips. Anchor the band behind you. Bend over and pull the band forward between your knees, locking your hands in place around it. Take a couple of steps forward and feel how the band wants to pull you back. Keep your back straight and allow your hips to go up to the maximum flexion point for your flexibility. Then push yourself upright by using your feet, still keeping your back straight (Barbara M, 2019).
- Hip thrust: See this exercise in the first workout program.
- Chest press: See the discussion in the first program, for the routine on day one.
- Arnold press: See earlier discussions.
- Standing wide row: An alternative to the rowing exercise discussed earlier is to stand with one foot a few steps in front of the other. The forward leg should be the opposite of your working arm. Pull the band towards you while rotating your torso and keeping your elbow flared out (*Alternative Exercises Row*, n.d.).
- Torso rotation: See earlier discussions.

- Side plank reach: See earlier discussions.
- Mountain climber: See earlier discussions.

Day Three

The exercises should be performed as a circuit, starting with the first exercise and ending with the last one, before going back to number one. The time for the workout should be about 36 minutes.

- Push-up: See earlier discussions.
- Glute bridge: See earlier discussions.
- Bicycle crunch: See earlier discussions.
- Banded squat: See earlier discussions.
- Lateral walk: See earlier discussions.
- Band pull-apart: Stand or sit up straight with a band looped around your hands. Pull your hands away from each other as far as you can and hold the position for a couple of seconds. Squeeze your shoulder blades together while doing this. You can also try to pull diagonally instead of in a straight line, as well as holding your arms at different heights to change the degree of difficulty (Coachmag, n.d.).
- Overhead press: See earlier discussions.
- Biceps curl: See earlier discussions.
- Bent-over rear delt fly: See earlier discussions.

Four Workouts per Week Program

Day One

The exercises should be performed as supersets, consisting of three sets with 10 to 12 repetitions each. Make sure the seventh repetition becomes challenging. The workout should take about 40 minutes.

- Band-assisted pull-up: See earlier discussions.
- Push-up: See earlier discussions.
- Arnold press: See earlier discussions.
- Face pull: See earlier discussions.
- High curl: Anchor the band in front of you at eye level. Hold the ends and step back until you can feel the tension in the band. Pull the band towards you, bending your elbows at a 90-degree angle and keeping your back straight and your core muscles tight (Rubberbanditz, 2019)
- Overhead extension: See earlier discussions.
- High-low chop: See earlier discussions.
- Mountain climber: See earlier discussions.

Day Two

The exercises should be performed as supersets, consisting of three sets with 10 to 12 repetitions each. Make sure the seventh repetition becomes challenging. The workout should take about 40 minutes.

- Single-leg bench squat: See earlier discussions.
- Split squat: See earlier discussions.
- Banded squat: See earlier discussions.
- Mountain climber: See earlier discussions.
- Clamshell: See earlier discussions.
- Lateral walk: See earlier discussions.

Day Three

The exercises should be performed as supersets, consisting of three sets with 12 to 15 repetitions each. Make sure the tenth repetition becomes challenging. The workout should take about 40 minutes.

- Standing wide row: See earlier discussions.
- Overhead press: See earlier discussions.
- Chest press: See earlier discussions.
- Band pull-apart: See earlier discussions.
- Biceps curl: See earlier discussions.
- Triceps kickback: Stand on a longish resistance band and bend forward from the waist. Hold the ends of the band in your hands and pull backward while in the bent position, reaching back as far as possible. For variety, you can try it with one arm at a time (BIQ Band Training, 2020).
- Lateral raise: See earlier discussions.
- High plank row: See earlier discussions.

Day Four

The exercises should be performed as supersets, consisting of three sets with 12 to 15 repetitions each. Make sure the tenth repetition becomes challenging. The workout should take about 40 minutes.

- Lying abduction: See earlier discussions.
- Hip thrust: See earlier discussions.
- Banded squat: See earlier discussions.
- Band-assisted pistol squats: See earlier discussions.
- Pull-through: See earlier discussions.
- Low-high chop: See earlier discussions.

Beginner Five or Six Day Workout

Are you ready to start your journey to fitness?

Keep the general background and guiding of the previous chapters in mind and listen to your body. While exercises should be challenging, they should not cause pain. Remember to warm-up properly and stretch and cool down afterward.

Prioritize the full range of motion in all exercises. Do it slower but all the way instead of trying to rush through the routine. Remember, this is dedicated time to yourself.

Adapt your goal to your current reality. Things that might have mattered to you twenty years ago are not so important anymore. Give yourself realistic reasons to show up for your home workout, and motivation will never be a problem, derailing your vision of a healthier and happier you.

Invest some time in learning meditation or tai chi, if you are so inclined. These mind exercises can be a great aid in visualizing the road ahead as well as the end result.

New experiences take time before you can get into your comfort zone, where they are easy. Give yourself that time and be kind to yourself; you're worth it.

Day One

This routine focuses on the lower body. The exercises should be performed as supersets, consisting of three sets with 12 to 15 repetitions each. Make sure the tenth repetition becomes challenging. The workout should take about 15 to 20 minutes with minimal breaks.

- Single-leg high extension: Anchor your band at waist height and feel it pull taut. Lift one knee as high as possible while pulling away from the anchor. For variety, you can lift the foot on the ground onto your toes at the same time (The Prehab Guys, n.d.).
- Pull-through: See earlier discussions.
- Glute bridge: See earlier discussions.
- Lying abduction: See earlier discussions.

Day Two

This routine is for the upper body. The exercises should be performed as supersets, consisting of three sets with 12 to 15 repetitions each. Make sure the tenth repetition becomes challenging. The workout should take about 15 to 20 minutes with minimal breaks.

- Bent-over row: See earlier discussions.
- Chest press: See earlier discussions.
- Overhead press: See earlier discussions.
- Side plank reach: See earlier discussions.

Day Three

This routine is for the lower body again. The exercises should be performed as supersets, consisting of three sets with 12 to 15 repetitions each. Make sure the seventh repetition becomes challenging. The workout should take about 15 to 20 minutes with minimal breaks.

- Single-leg deadlift: See earlier discussions.

- Split squat: See earlier discussions.
- Hip thrust: See earlier discussions.
- Bicycle crunch: See earlier discussions.

Day Four

An upper body routine today. The exercises should be performed as supersets, consisting of three sets with 12 to 15 repetitions each. Make sure the seventh repetition becomes challenging. The workout should take about 15 to 20 minutes with minimal breaks.

- Kneeling pull-down: See earlier discussions.
- Push-up: See earlier discussions.
- Arnold press: See earlier discussions.
- Side plank row: See earlier discussions.

Day Five

Today it is the turn of the full body. The exercises should be performed as a circuit, starting with the first exercise and ending with the last one, before going back to number one. The time for the workout should be about 20 minutes.

- Bent-over rear delt fly: See earlier discussions.
- Banded squat: See earlier discussions.
- Mountain climber: See earlier discussions.
- Overhead press: See earlier discussions.
- Hip raise: See earlier discussions.

Day Six

The whole body will again be exercised today. The exercises should be performed as supersets, consisting of three sets with 12 to 15 repetitions each. Make sure the seventh repetition becomes challenging. The workout should take about 15 to 20 minutes with minimal breaks.

- Chest press: See earlier discussions.
- Split squat: See earlier discussions.
- Face pull: See earlier discussions.
- High-low chop: See earlier discussions.

Advanced Five or Six Day Workout

Congratulations on getting this far, if you mastered the beginner routine first. You have progressed well on your way to a healthy, happy, and physically easier future.

For more advanced readers who start here, this program should provide enough of a challenge to get you moving. Use it as an example to put your own program together as it suits you.

Day One

These exercises are for the lower body. The exercises should be performed as supersets, consisting of three sets with 10 to 12 repetitions each. Make sure the tenth repetition becomes challenging. The workout should take about 40 to 50 minutes, with minimal breaks.

- Single-leg hip extension: See earlier discussions.
- Pull-through: See earlier discussions.
- Skater squats: See earlier discussions.
- Quadruped kickback: See earlier discussions.
- Glute bridge: See earlier discussions.
- Hip thrust: See earlier discussions.
- Banded squat: See earlier discussions.

- Torso rotation: See earlier discussions.

Day Two

Today we exercise the upper body. The exercises should be performed as supersets, consisting of three sets with 12 to 15 repetitions each. Make sure the tenth repetition becomes challenging. The workout should take about 40 to 50 minutes, with minimal breaks.

- Bent-over row: See earlier discussions.
- Chest press: See earlier discussions.
- Overhead press: See earlier discussions.
- Straight-arm pulldown: For variety on the arm pulldown exercise discussed earlier, you can keep your arms straight instead of bending them at the elbows. You could insert something like a light wooden rod in the loops of the band and place your hands at the ends of the rod instead of in the middle. That will keep your elbows wider and engage even more muscles (Rubberbanditz, 2019).
- Triceps press-down: To change the degree of difficulty from the exercise as discussed earlier, you could do this one arm at a time while keeping your core muscles tight and your back and ribcage straight (Showman, 2017).
- High curl: See earlier discussions.
- Mountain climber: See earlier discussions.
- Side plank reach: See earlier discussions.

Day Three

It is the lower body's turn again. The exercises should be performed as supersets, consisting of three sets with 12 to 15 repetitions each. Make sure the seventh repetition becomes challenging. The workout should take about 40 to 50 minutes, with minimal breaks.

- Single-leg deadlift: See earlier discussions.
- Split squat: See earlier discussions.
- Single-leg bench squat: See earlier discussions.
- Clamshell: See earlier discussions.
- Lateral walk: See earlier discussions.
- Hip thrust: See earlier discussions.
- Psoas march: See earlier discussions.
- Bicycle crunch: See earlier discussions.

Day Four

Time for the upper body to get a chance again. The exercises should be performed as supersets, consisting of three sets with 10 to 12 repetitions each. Make sure the seventh repetition becomes challenging. The workout should take about 40 to 50 minutes, with minimal breaks.

- Kneeling pull-down: See earlier discussions.
- Push-up: See earlier discussions.
- Arnold press: See earlier discussions.
- Band-assisted pull-up: See earlier discussions.
- Low biceps curl: Instead of standing in front of the band when pulling it towards you, you can lie down on the floor and pull the band from a low anchor. Keep your knees bent and your back and hips flat on the floor (Rubberbanditz, 2019).

- Overhead extension: See earlier discussions.
- Pec Fly: Also known as the chest fly exercise. See earlier discussions.
- Side Plank row: See earlier discussions.

Day Five

Today it is the turn of the full body. The exercises should be performed as a circuit, starting with the first exercise and ending with the last one, before going back to number one. The time for the workout should be about 36 minutes.

- Bent-over rear delt fly: See earlier discussions.
- Push-up: See earlier discussions.
- Banded squat: See earlier discussions.
- Glute bridge: See earlier discussions.
- Mountain climber: See earlier discussions.
- Overhead press: See earlier discussions.
- Biceps curl: See earlier discussions.
- Skater squats: See earlier discussions.
- Hip raise: See earlier discussions.

Day Six

The whole body will again be exercised today. The exercises should be performed as supersets, consisting of three sets with 12 to 15 repetitions each. Make sure the seventh repetition becomes challenging. The workout should take about 40 to 50 minutes with minimal breaks.

- Chest press: See earlier discussions.
- Split squat: See earlier discussions.
- Pallof press: Anchor your band firmly at shoulder height. Hold the end of the band in both hands against

your chest. You can either stand or kneel, although the kneeling version is slightly more difficult. Step away from the anchor far enough that you can feel the band pulling you back. Straighten your arms towards the anchor and engage your core muscles to stay upright with a straight back. Resist the band's attempts to get your torso to twist. Hold the position for as long as possible before relaxing (Coachmag, n.d.).

- Band-assisted pistol squats: See earlier discussions.
- Hip hinge: See earlier discussions.
- Single-leg bench squat: See earlier discussions.
- Face pull: See earlier discussions.
- High-low chop: See earlier discussions.

Your new habit and routines are started. Keep the momentum going, do not stop now. Your body and mind will thank you every day for the decision you took when you picked this book up, to invest time and effort in your health.

It is all about vitality and living your senior years with vigor. It is being able to experience the fullest range of functional movement possible given your specific situation.

Conclusion

Are you as excited as I am for you to start on the beautiful and rewarding road to a healthier, fitter, and happier version of yourself than you've ever been?

We started this journey of discovery looking at the what and the why of resistance bands. I told you a little bit about myself and my amazing experiences with exercise, as well as my passion for helping others to discover the same satisfaction and live their dream lives.

We looked at the benefits of exercise in general and uncovered its power and potential to prevent and heal certain illnesses and medical conditions. You learned all the reasons why resistance band training is an excellent way to harness the healing and rejuvenating properties of regular exercise.

I also introduced you to your new exercise companion, your set of resistance bands. Together we looked at the different types of bands available, the options they offer, and accessories that make them even more versatile. We briefly looked at some resistance exercises specific to golfers because there are so many seniors enjoying the sport. Golf is only one example of how bands can improve any game and prevent injuries.

You now know exactly what to do and what not to do for the best results. You have practiced some of the movements with me and experienced for yourself how much better you feel. You have seen for yourself how different exercises go together and complement each other for a whole body benefit. You have also acquired the know-how to compile your own workout routines to suit your circumstances and preferences perfectly.

A Final Piece of Advice

You have all the right knowledge and tools in your hands now, but it remains up to you to apply them to your life. You will not reap the success you desire if you do not make a commitment to yourself or a training partner to show up for regular workouts.

Your life is in your hands, and the choice is yours. Take the right decision and make today the first day of the new *You*!

It has been great fun to help you down this road of discovery. Thank you for allowing me to share my passion and some of my knowledge and experience. My biggest reward will be knowing that it transformed your life. Kindly leave a positive review of this book to let me know how it is working for you and so others can experience the improvements of having their own "fitness bible" on demand.

References

8fit Team. (n.d.). *8 Benefits of Resistance Bands and Two Workouts*. 8fit. https://8fit.com/fitness/resistance-band-benefits-and-workouts/

Alexander. (2011, August 12). *Don't Hold Your Breath - Suffocation Will Affect your Workouts Negatively*. Fitzness.Com. http://www.fitzness.com/blog/dont-hold-your-breath-suffocation-will-affect-your-workouts-negatively/

Alternative Exercises Row. (n.d.). Your Body Programme. https://www.yourbodyprogramme.com/alternative-exercises-row

Alzheimer's Society UK. (n.d.). *Physical exercise and dementia*. Alzheimer's Society. https://www.alzheimers.org.uk/about-dementia/risk-factors-and-prevention/physical-exercise#:~:text=Combining%20the%20results%20of%2011

Amazon. (n.d.). *Grebest Heavy Duty Resistance Band, Pull UP Assist Bands Workout Resistance Bands for Body Stretching Powerlifting Mobility Single Band or Set*. Amazon. https://www.amazon.com/Grebest-Resistance-Powerlifting-Stretching-Weightlifting/dp/B079DNQTVT/ref=asc_df_B079DNQTVT/?tag=hyprod-20&linkCode=df0&hvadid=309821907754&hvpos=&hvnetw=g&hvrand=7597129508290966102&hvpone=&hvptwo=&hvqmt=&hvdev=c&hvdvcmdl=&

hvlocint=&hvlocphy=9033326&hvtargid=pla-599317122411&psc=1

Amazon. (2020). *Amazon.com : RENRANRING Resistance Bands Set, Exercise Bands with Stackable Workout Bands, Door Anchor Attachment, Handles, Legs Ankle Straps, Carry Bag, Gym Equipment for Home (Set of 13) (Black) : Sports & Outdoors*. Amazon. https://www.amazon.com/RENRANRING-Resistance-Stackable-Attachment-Equipment/dp/B08134VTJ6

Amazon Valeofit Store. (2020). *Valeo: Recovery*. Amazon. https://www.amazon.com/stores/page/692DC80A-844C-4D4E-B825-E950AE4275C8?ingress=2&visitId=c00a56a1-4f3d-4d1c-ada3-16ac48ea1907&ref_=ast_bln

Amazon.com : SUPERPUMP BFR BANDS | Simple + Effective Quick-Release Straps for Blood Flow Restriction Training and Kaatsu Style Workouts | Arms : Sports & Outdoors. (2020). Amazon. https://www.amazon.com/Superpump-Kaatsu-inspired-Training-Restriction-Maximum/dp/B01N45Z84Y

Andersen, C. (2014, July 10). *47 Crazy-Fun Plank Variations*. Greatest. https://greatist.com/move/plank-variations-for-core-strength#intermediate

Arana, J. (2019, March 29). *3 Ways to Perform Assisted Pull Ups - wikiHow Fitness*. Www.Wikihow.Fitness.

https://www.wikihow.fitness/Perform-Assisted-Pull-Ups

Arnold Press - How To Do It. (n.d.). Move More Eat Better! http://www.exercise-guide-to-lose-weight.com/arnold-press.html

Atemi Sports. (2019, August 12). 15 Mini Resistance Band Ab Exercises for a Rock-Solid Core. Atemi Sports. https://www.atemi-sports.com/mini-resistance-band-ab-exercises/

Barbara M. (2019, August 7). Featured Exercise: Banded Pull-Throughs. Barbell Strength. http://barbell-strength.com/banded-pullthrough/

Barber, E. (2018, December 11). Get Fit with a Resistance Band. Archery 360. https://www.archery360.com/2018/12/11/get-fit-with-a-resistance-band/#:~:text=Start%20by%20folding%20the%20band

Bentley, A. (2016, December 3). Tip: Use Bands for Lateral Raises. T NATION. https://www.t-nation.com/training/tip-use-bands-for-lateral-raises

BfR Professional. (2018). Blood Flow Restriction Training- A complete guide. BfR Professional. https://bfrpro.com/pages/blood-flow-restriction-training

BIQ Band Training. (2020, May 3). Hip Thrust With Resistance Band. BiqBandTraning.Com.

https://biqbandtraining.com/hip-thrust-with-resistance-band/?v=7516fd43adaa

Biswas, C. (2018, April 25). *18 Best Resistance Band Exercises - Full Body Workouts.* STYLECRAZE. https://www.stylecraze.com/articles/resistance-band-exercises/#resistance-band-exercises-for-the-abscore

Bowden, J. (2015, October 9). *6 exercises using resistance bands for more distance.* Golf WRX. http://www.golfwrx.com/329714/6-exercises-using-resistance-bands-for-more-distance/

Brathwaite, P. (2018, February 9). *How to Perfect the Banded Curl.* Muscle & Fitness. https://www.muscleandfitness.com/workouts/arm-exercises/how-perfect-banded-curl-massive-biceps/

Cadman, B. (2020, January 24). *10 exercises to strengthen the lower back.* Www.Medicalnewstoday.Com. https://www.medicalnewstoday.com/articles/323204#lower-back-rotational-stretches

Callaway, M. (2018, December 7). *6 Psoas March Variations You Likely Haven't Tried Before |.* Meghan Callaway. http://www.meghancallawayfitness.com/my-blog/6-psoas-march-variations-you-likely-havent-tried-before/

Carpenter, H. (2020, May 21). *Use This Simple Progression to Work into a Pistol Squat.* Outside Online.

https://www.outsideonline.com/2412982/how-do-pistol-squat

Chowdhury, M. H. (2019, September 22). *Best Resistance Bands For Seniors, And People Of Any Age For Bodybuilding*. Fitness of Body | Health and Fitness Tips, Healthy Food Habits Etc. https://www.fitnessofbody.com/2019/09/best-resistance-bands-for-seniors-any-age.html

Coachmag. (n.d.). *How To Do The Pallof Press*. Coach. https://www.coachmag.co.uk/core-exercises/7392/how-to-do-the-pallof-press#:~:text=Engage%20your%20core%20and%20press

Collins, R. (2012, March 29). *Exercise, Depression, and the Brain*. Healthline. https://www.healthline.com/health/depression/exercise#:~:text=They%20help%20relieve%20pain%20and

Cordeau, B. (n.d.). *Lat Pulldown Loop Band*. Skimble. https://www.skimble.com/exercises/41947-lat-pulldown-loop-band-how-to-do-exercise

Creveling, M. (2020, June 18). *Can You Build Muscle Without Lifting Weights?* Shape. https://www.shape.com/fitness/workouts/bodyweight-training/build-muscle-bodyweight-exercises

Crowley, G. (2016, April 5). *Pilates – the importance of controlled movement*. Health Through Harmony.

https://www.healththroughharmony.ie/pilates-the-importance-of-controlled-movement/

Cruz, N. (2019, June 7). *10 Ways to Get Stronger Without Lifting Weights*. LIVESTRONG.COM. https://www.livestrong.com/article/335541-ten-ways-to-get-stronger-without-lifting-weights/

De Pietro, M. (2019, January 22). *Trapezius: Muscle pain, stretches, and home remedies*. Www.Medicalnewstoday.Com. https://www.medicalnewstoday.com/articles/324251

Dearden, K. (2017, December 13). *What are Therapeutic Resistance Bands?* Newcastle Sports Injury Clinic. https://www.newcastlesportsinjury.co.uk/what-are-therapeutic-resistance-bands/

Desertcart. (n.d.). *Shop brand renranring Online at Low Price in Botswana at botswana.desertcart.com*. Botswana. https://botswana.desertcart.com/brands/brand-renranring

Dick's Pro Tips. (2019, April 12). *Five Upper Body Resistance Band Exercises*. PRO TIPS by DICK'S Sporting Goods. https://protips.dickssportinggoods.com/sports-and-activities/exercise-and-fitness/five-upper-body-resistance-band-exercises

Dotfit. (n.d.). *Tennis Watcher*. Dotfit. https://www.dotfit.com/sites/63/images/articles/Exercise%20PDFs/Tennis%20Watcher.pdf

EDX USA. (n.d.). *Resistance*. EDX.
https://edxusa.com/collections/resistance

EFM Healthclubs. (2018, October 19). *6 Benefits of
Abdominal Workouts*. EFM Health Clubs.
https://efm.net.au/benefits-of-abdominal-workouts/

Eisinger, A. (2019, November 8). *13 Super Effective
Exercises That Work Your Arms, Back, and
Shoulders*. SELF.
https://www.self.com/gallery/arm-sculpting-
slideshow

Fairview. (n.d.). *Neck Exercises: Head Lifts*. Fairview.
https://www.fairview.org/sitecore/content/Fairview/
Home/Patient-
Education/Articles/English/n/e/c/k/_/Neck_Exercise
s_Head_Lifts_85975

Fanelli, L. (n.d.). *How to Use Resistance Bands for Strength
Training*. Tomsofmaine.
https://www.tomsofmaine.com/good-
matters/healthy-feeling/how-to-use-resistance-
bands-for-strength-
training#:~:text=Simply%20stand%20on%the%2
0band

Fetters, K. A. (2016, September 28). *Why Range of Motion
Matters for Your Strength Training Goals*. Life by
Daily Burn.
https://dailyburn.com/life/fitness/strength-training-
range-of-motion/

Fetters, K. A. (2019, December 27). *Why You Should Try the Windmill Exercise (and How to Do it)*. Openfit. https://www.openfit.com/windmill-exercise

Fit Carrots. (n.d.). *Core - Side Bends with Long Resistance Band*. FIT CARROTS | Premium Fitness Tools For Functional and Regeneration Training. https://www.fitcarrots.com/exercise/long-resistance-bands/core-side-bends-with-long-resistance-band/

Fitness Australia. (2018). *Resistance training – health benefits*. Better Health. https://www.betterhealth.vic.gov.au/health/healthyliving/resistance-training-health-benefits

Fort Healthcare. (2019, January 10). *Hand & Wrist Stretches for Computer/Smartphone Users*. Fort HealthCare. https://www.forthealthcare.com/hand-and-wrist-stretches-for-computer-and-smartphone-users/#:~:text=ceiling%20wrist%20stretch-

Freytag, C. (2014, July 12). *How To Use A Figure 8 Band*. Get Healthy U | Chris Freytag. https://gethealthyu.com/how-to-use-a-figure-8-band/

Garage Gym Reviews. (n.d.). *Best Tube Resistance Bands for 2020*. Garagegymreviews. https://www.garagegymreviews.com/best-tube-resistance-bands

Giacobbe, L. (2019, September 25). *How older adults can recover from exercise injuries*. Kendalathome. https://www.kendalathome.org/blog/bid/314169/how-older-adults-can-recover-from-exercise-injuries

Gomez, A. (2017, August 11). *This Tiny Tweak Will Take Your Mountain Climbers To The Next Level.* Women's Health. https://www.womenshealthmag.com/fitness/a19916 561/fitgif-friday-mini-band-mountain-climber/

Gunsmith Fitness. (n.d.). *Hip Circles 101: Everything You Need to Know About This Unique Training Device.* Gunsmith Fitness. https://gunsmithfitness.com/blogs/news/hip-circles-101

Hagstrom, A. D., Marshall, P. W., Halaki, M., & Hackett, D. A. (2019). The Effect of Resistance Training in Women on Dynamic Strength and Muscular Hypertrophy: A Systematic Review with Meta-analysis. *Sports Medicine (Auckland, N.Z.), 50,* 10.1007/s40279-019-01247–x. https://doi.org/10.1007/s40279-019-01247-x

Harwood, R. (2018, March 22). *Resistance Band's with Handles VS without Handles.* Fitness Health. https://fitnesshealth.co/blogs/fitness/resistance-bands-with-handles-vs-without-handles

Health Benefits Of Physical Activity. (2019). MedicineNet. https://www.medicinenet.com/script/main/art.asp?ar ticlekey=10074

Healthwise Incorporated. (2020, March 2). *Tennis Elbow | Senior Health Services.* Hhcseniorservices.Org. https://hhcseniorservices.org/health-wellness/health-resources/health-library/detail?id=hw225372&lang=en-us

HEB. (2020). *Protein Building Blocks*. H-E-B | No Store Does More. https://www.heb.com/static-page/article-template/Protein-Building-Blocks

Herman, D. (2017, October 16). *Benefits of Resistance Bands in Golf*. Super Flex® Fitness. https://www.superflexfitness.com/benefits-of-resistance-bands-in-golf/

Hoffman, K. (2020, April 3). *9 Best Resistance Band Chest Exercises To Do At Home*. NOOB GAINS. https://noobgains.com/resistance-band-chest-exercises/

Iliades, C. (2019, May 13). *The Benefits of Strength and Weight Training | Everyday Health*. EverydayHealth.Com. https://www.everydayhealth.com/fitness/add-strength-training-to-your-workout.aspx

Jay, J. (2010, September 30). *Exercise Order - How To Arrange Exercises In Your Workout*. A Workout Routine. https://www.aworkoutroutine.com/exercise-order/

Jewell, T. (2018, September 25). *Diaphragmatic Breathing and Its Benefits*. Healthline. https://www.healthline.com/health/diaphragmatic-breathing#benefits

Kamau, C. (2020, August 10). *Calorie Deficit But Not Losing Weight: What's The Culprit Behind It?* Weight Loss Blog - BetterMe.

https://betterme.world/articles/calorie-deficit-but-not-losing-weight/#:~:text=Yes%2C%20it%20is.

Kassel, G. (2019, May 23). *How to Use Resistance Bands— Because You Know You Don't *Really* Know.* Shape. https://www.shape.com/fitness/tips/how-use-resistance-bands

Kelly, E. (2015, October 22). *What You Need to Know About Anaerobic Exercise.* Healthline; Healthline Media. https://www.healthline.com/health/fitness-exercise/anaerobic-exercise#benefits

Kelso, T. (n.d.). *The Top 5 Exercises to Strengthen Your Neck.* Breaking Muscle. https://breakingmuscle.com/fitness/the-top-5-exercises-to-strengthen-your-neck

Kendola, A. (2020, July 23). *8 lower back stretches for flexibility and pain relief.* Www.Medicalnewstoday.Com. https://www.medicalnewstoday.com/articles/lower-back-stretches#knee-to-chest

Kilroy, D. S. (2014). *Exercise and Eating Healthy.* Healthline. https://www.healthline.com/health/fitness-exercise-eating-healthy

Knopf, K. (2010). *Healthy shoulder handbook : 100 exercises for treating and preventing frozen shoulder, rotator cuff and other common injuries.* Ulysses Press.

Kwon, Y. S., & Kravitz, L. (2019). *How Do Muscles Grow?* Unm.Edu. https://www.unm.edu/~lkravitz/Article%20folder/musclesgrowLK.html

Letsfit. (n.d.). *Fitness Accessories - Letsfit.* Www.Letsfit.Com. Retrieved October 20, 2020, from https://www.letsfit.com/product-list/110/Fitness_Accessories

Level, B., Sydney, 499 Kent St, & Email, N. S. W. 2000 A. +61 2 9267 5487. (2017, November 13). *15 Essential Foods You Need on a Fat Loss Diet - Ultimate Performance.* Ultimate Performance Sydney. https://up-australia.com/tips/15-essential-foods-need-transformation-diet/

Lori Michiel Fitness, Inc. (n.d.). *Choosing and using resistance bands in workouts for seniors.* Lori Michiel Fitness, Inc. https://lorimichielfitness.com/resources/exercise-resistance-bands/

Lugo, J. (2017, August 15). *Lower Body Exercise: Skaters With A Mini-Band.* JLFITNESSMIAMI. https://juanlugofitness.com/lower-body-exercise-skaters-with-a-mini-band/

Lux Fitness. (n.d.). *Premium Booty Resistance Band Set.* Lux Retails. Retrieved October 20, 2020, from https://luxretails.com/products/hip-resistance-band-set

Marcin, A. (2018, February 12). *Tight Calves: Stretches, Treatment, Prevention, Causes, and More.* Healthline. https://www.healthline.com/health/tight-calves#causes

Mateo, A. (2017, October 9). *Legit Resistance Band Ab Workout.* Greatist. https://greatist.com/fitness/resistance-band-core-exercises-massy-arias#exercises

Matt. (n.d.). *How To Anchor Your Resistance Bands At Home: Easy and Cheap.* Home Gym Resource. https://homegymresource.com/how-to-anchor-your-resistance-bands-at-home-easy-and-cheap/

Maximum Training Solutions. (2016, July 20). *5 Variations of the Mini Band Sidestep.* Maximum Training Solutions -. http://www.maximumtrainingsolutions.com/5-variations-of-the-mini-band-sidestep/

Mayo Clinic. (2016). *Osteoporosis - Symptoms and causes.* Mayo Clinic. https://www.mayoclinic.org/diseases-conditions/osteoporosis/symptoms-causes/syc-20351968

Mayo Clinic. (2018, December 18). *What you need to know about exercise and chronic disease.* Mayo Clinic. https://www.mayoclinic.org/healthy-lifestyle/fitness/in-depth/exercise-and-chronic-disease/art-20046049#:~:text=Regular%20exercise%20can%20help%20insulin

Men's Health. (2011, May 4). *You MUST Try This Ab-Blasting Exercise!* Men's Health. https://www.menshealth.com/fitness/a19529948/side-plank-and-row/

Merriam-Webster. (2011). *Definition of STRENGTH TRAINING.* Merriam-Webster.Com. https://www.merriam-webster.com/dictionary/strength%20training

Mirafit. (n.d.). *Top 8 Resistance Band Shoulder Exercises | Mirafit.* Mirafit.Co.Uk. https://mirafit.co.uk/blog/best-shoulder-exercises-using-resistance-bands/#:~:text=Tie%20the%20resistance%20band%20to

Mulrooney, M. (2011, July 8). *Figure 8 Resistance Band Exercises.* SportsRec. https://www.sportsrec.com/412995-figure-8-resistance-band-exercises.html

Murthi, A. M., & Ramirez, M. A. (2012). *Shoulder dislocation in older patients poses different challenges in diagnosis, treatment.* ScienceDaily. https://www.sciencedaily.com/releases/2012/10/121004134837.htm

National Posture Institute. (2014, March). *Why Postural Alignment is Important in Exercise Progression.* Www.Npionline.Org. https://www.npionline.org/articles/why-postural-alignment-is-important-in-exercise-progression

New Heights Physical Therapy. (n.d.). *The Three Phases of Healing | Portland OR & Vancouver WA*. New Heights Physical Therapy Plus in Portland OR Vancouver WA. https://www.newheightstherapy.com/phases-of-healing/

Newhouse, R. (2013, July 30). *The benefits of proper breathing during exercise*. MyNetDiary. https://www.mynetdiary.com/the-benefits-of-proper-breathing-during-exercise.html

NIAGARA LUTHERAN HEALTH FOUNDATION. (2016). *5 Benefits of Exercise for Seniors and Aging Adults | The GreenFields Continuing Care Community | Lancaster, NY*. Thegreenfields.Org. https://thegreenfields.org/5-benefits-exercise-seniors-aging-adults/

No Foam Roller? No Problem! Try These Alternatives! | ISSA. (n.d.). Www.Issaonline.Com. https://www.issaonline.com/blog/index.cfm/2020/no-foam-roller-no-problem-try-these-alternatives

Nunez, K. (2018, August 16). *Need a Leg Press Alternative? 5 to Try*. Healthline. https://www.healthline.com/health/leg-press-alternative#resistance-bands

Patricie K. (n.d.). *Lying Band Back Fly*. Skimble. https://www.skimble.com/exercises/37666-lying-band-back-fly-how-to-do-exercise

Pedemonte, S. (2020, October 1). *How to Perform a Torso Twist*. Your House Fitness. https://www.yourhousefitness.com/blog/how-to-perform-the-torso-twist

Perfect Peach Athletics. (n.d.). *Perfect Peach Athletics - The #1 Fitness Brand for Women*. Perfect Peach Athletics. https://perfectpeachathletics.com/

Physioworks. (n.d.). *Exercise equipment – Physio Works*. https://physioworks.com.au/product-category/exercise-equipment/

Picincu, A. (2020, March 27). *Lawn Mowers and Back Exercise*. LIVESTRONG.COM. https://www.livestrong.com/article/336466-lawn-mowers-back-exercise/

Pridgett, T. (2019, June 15). *Burn Fat With This Cardio-Strengthening Bodyweight Exercise You Can Do Anywhere*. POPSUGAR Fitness. https://www.popsugar.com/fitness/How-Do-Resistance-Band-Sprints-46255833

Quinn, E. (2008, November 13). *How to Perform the Sit and Reach Flexibility Test*. Verywell Fit; Verywellfit. https://www.verywellfit.com/sit-and-reach-flexibility-test-3120279

Quinn, E. (2020, April 28). *What Exercises Help With ACL Rehabilitation?* Verywell Health. https://www.verywellhealth.com/acl-surgery-rehab-exercises-3120748

Rehabbing Sports Injuries with Resistance Bands. (2018, December 15). Prohealthcareproducts.Com. https://www.prohealthcareproducts.com/blog/rehabbing-sports-injuries-with-resistance-bands/

Resistance Band Lat Pulldown. (n.d.). Exercise. https://www.exercise.com/exercises/resistance-band-lat-pulldown

Resistance Band Lateral Raise. (n.d.). Exercise. https://www.exercise.com/exercises/resistance-band-lateral-raise

Rubberbanditz. (2019, February 6). *Chest Exercises with Resistance Bands*. Www.Rubberbanditz.Com. https://www.rubberbanditz.com/blog/chest-exercises-with-resistance-bands/

Rusin, J. (2017, June 14). *5 Ways To Make Face Pulls Even Better*. T NATION. https://www.t-nation.com/training/5-ways-to-make-face-pulls-even-better

Salyer, J. (2016, April 14). *Bridge Exercise: 5 Fun and Challenging Variations*. Healthline. https://www.healthline.com/health/fitness-exercise/glute-bridge-variations

Schrift, D. (2014). *How to Start With Exercises For The Elderly? Read on...* Elder gym®. https://eldergym.com/exercises-for-the-elderly/

Set for Set. (2017). *7 Rotator Cuff Resistance Band Exercises for Shoulder Rehab & Strength*. SET FOR

SET. https://www.setforset.com/blogs/news/7-rotator-cuff-resistance-bands-exercises-for-rehab-prehab-and-strengthening

Set for Set. (2019, May 18). *What Size Resistance Bands Should I Get? Your Guide to Buying Bands.* SET FOR SET. https://www.setforset.com/blogs/news/what-size-resistance-bands-should-i-buy

Sheppard, L. M. (2014). *How latex is made - material, production process, making, history, used, processing, components, composition.* Madehow.Com. http://www.madehow.com/Volume-3/Latex.html

Showman, N. (2017, September 14). *4 Resistance Band Exercises to Build Tricep Strength.* Muscle & Strength. https://www.muscleandstrength.com/articles/4-resistance-band-tricep-exercises

Simple Fitness Solutions. (n.d.). *Guidelines for exercise bands and exercise balls.* Simplefitnesssolutions. https://www.simplefitnesssolutions.com/resources/Guidelines.htm

Skimble. (n.d.). *Dumbbell Fly on Ball.* Skimble. https://www.skimble.com/exercises/2239-dumbbell-fly-on-ball-how-to-do-exercise

Snape, J. (2015, July 15). *Ectomorph, Endomorph And Mesomorph: How To Train For Your Body Type.* Coach; Coach.

https://www.coachmag.co.uk/lifestyle/4511/ectomor
ph-endomorph-or-mesomorph-what-is-your-body-
type

SoCal Health. (n.d.). *SoCal Health Group*. SoCal Health.
https://socalhealthgroup.com

Soto, P. (2018, February 8). *The Single Leg Deadlift with a
Resistance Band version*. Sports and Martial Arts in
the United States and the Modern World.
https://sportsandmartialarts.com/single-leg-deadlift-
resistance-band-challenge/

Spark People. (n.d.). *Lying Abduction with Band Exercise
Demonstration*. SparkPeople.
https://www.sparkpeople.com/resource/exercises.as
p?exercise=1

Starwood Sports. (n.d.). *Resistance Loop Band Exercise
Guide*. Starwood Sports.
https://uk.starwoodsports.com/pages/resistance-
loop-band-exercise-guide

Sworkit Wellness. (n.d.). *Resistance Band Overhead Press*.
Sworkit | At Home Workout and Fitness Plans.
https://sworkit.com/exercise/resistance-band-
overhead-press-
2#:~:text=Stand%20on%20your%20resistance%20b
and

Taraniuk, L. (2019, July 22). *The importance of breathing
during workouts*. Totalbalancehf.
https://www.totalbalancehf.com/single-
post/2019/07/01/The-importance-of-breathing-

during-
workouts#:~:text=When%20you%20exercise%20an
d%20your

*The Definitive Guide to Resistance Bands and Workout
Bands*. (n.d.). WODFitters.
https://www.wodfitters.com/pages/the-definitive-
guide-to-resistance-bands-and-workout-bands

The Movement Fix. (2018, September 3). *Standing Banded
Row*. Movement Fix.
https://themovementfix.com/standing-banded-row/

The Prehab Guys. (n.d.). *Double Leg Hip Hinge With
Resistance Band*. **[P]Rehab**.
https://theprehabguys.com/vimeo-video/double-leg-
hip-hinge-with-resistance-band/

The right way to warm up and cool down. (2019, July 9).
Mayo Clinic. https://www.mayoclinic.org/healthy-
lifestyle/fitness/in-depth/exercise/art-
20045517#:~:text=A%20warmup%20gradually%20
revs%20up

Theraband. (n.d.). *About Us - TheraBand*.
Www.Theraband.Com. Retrieved October 20, 2020,
from https://www.theraband.com/about-us

Timco Rubber. (n.d.). *Rubber Extrusion Process, Extruded
Rubber Process*. Timcorubber.
https://www.timcorubber.com/rubber-
resources/rubber-extrusion-process/

Tinsley, G. (2017, October 1). *How to Improve Body Composition, Based on Science*. Healthline. https://www.healthline.com/nutrition/improve-body-composition#TOC_TITLE_HDR_4

Train With Me Fitness Inc. (n.d.). *Train Online Signup*. Trainonline. https://www.trainonline.com/reverse-band-woodchops-exercise

Tribe Fitness USA. (n.d.). *Resistance Bands*. Tribe Fitness. https://www.tribefitnessusa.com/collections/resistance-bands

University of Birmingham. (2018). *A lifetime of regular exercise slows down aging, study finds*. ScienceDaily. https://www.sciencedaily.com/releases/2018/03/180308143123.htm

University Orthopedics. (n.d.). *University Orthopedics - Foot and Ankle Exercises*. University Orthopedics. https://universityorthopedics.com/educational_resources/foot_exercises.html#:~:text=Ankle%20Stretch

Upham, B. (2018, April 6). *The Possible Way Strength Training Reduces Insulin Resistance | Everyday Health*. EverydayHealth.Com. https://www.everydayhealth.com/type-2-diabetes/treatment/mechanism-strength-training-can-help-reduce-insulin-resistance/

Victoria, A. (2016, October 25). *No clue how to foam roll? Watch this!* TODAY.Com.

https://www.today.com/health/foam-rolling-5-
minute-routine-stretch-your-body-t104297

Waehner, P. (2019, November 21). *Turn Your Exercise Ball
Into a Strength Training Machine*. Verywell Fit.
https://www.verywellfit.com/total-body-workout-
with-bands-on-the-ball-
1230909#:~:text=Chest%20Press

Watkins, W. (2014, December 19). *Fitness Fix:
Strengthening Your Pelvic-Floor Muscles*.
Experience Life.
https://experiencelife.com/article/fitness-fix-
strengthening-your-pelvic-floor-muscles/

WebMD. (n.d.). *What Is Trochanteric Bursitis?* WebMD.
Retrieved October 13, 2020, from
https://www.webmd.com/pain-
management/trochanteric-bursitis#1

WebMD. (2007). *Runner's Knee: What You Need to Know*.
WebMD; WebMD. https://www.webmd.com/pain-
management/knee-pain/runners-knee#1

Weight Loss Resources UK. (n.d.). *Upper Body Muscles*.
Weightloss Resources.
https://www.weightlossresources.co.uk/exercise/mu
scles/upper_body.htm

Weingart, H. M., & Kravitz, L. (2020). *Resistance Training
and Bone Mass*. Unm.Edu.
https://www.unm.edu/~lkravitz/Article%20folder/bo
nemass.html#:~:text=There%20is%20increasing%2
0emphasis%20on

What is Thermoplastic Rubber? (TPR). (2017, September 5). KMA SA Marketing. https://www.kmasa.co.za/thermoplastic-rubber-tpr/

Whatafit. (n.d.). *Whatafit - Shenzhen Yongming Wangluokeji Youxiangongsi.* Whatafit. http://www.whatafit.net/

Wheeler, T. (2019, December 18). *Slideshow: Benefits of Strength Training.* WebMD. https://www.webmd.com/fitness-exercise/ss/slideshow-benefits-strength

Williams, L. (2020, March 6). *Use the Quadruped Hip Extension to Build Better Glutes.* Verywell Fit. https://www.verywellfit.com/how-to-do-a-quadruped-hip-extension-4685857

Williamson, L. (2019, December 12). *Consistency Is The Most Important When Training For Muscle Growth.* Www.Womenshealth.Com.Au. https://www.womenshealth.com.au/consistency-most-important-factor-for-building-strength-muscle-growth-resistance-training

Winderl, A. M. (2017, June 27). *13 of the Best Exercises for Your Side Abs.* SELF. https://www.self.com/gallery/obliques-exercises

YMCA of the North. (n.d.). *Long-term benefits of regular exercise.* YMCA of the North. https://www.ymcanorth.org/blog/2017/04/04/5991/long_term_benefits_of_regular_exercise

Young, L. (2020, February 27). *4 Key Body Parts You Should Exercise Now*. Best Health Magazine Canada. https://www.besthealthmag.ca/best-you/fitness/main-body-parts-to-work-out/

Ziftex. (n.d.). *Products*. ZIFTEX. https://ziftex.com/collections/all

Images

Ashram, S. (n.d.). Seniors on yoga mats. In *Unsplash*. https://unsplash.com/photos/QgCl-pNkfPc

Canburn, L. (n.d.). Woman on fitness ball. In *Unsplash*. https://unsplash.com/photos/f4RBYsY2hxA

Cook, C. (nod-a). Shoulder stability is important for a golfer. In *Unsplash*. https://unsplash.com/photos/O_UZcIm2yqI

Cook, C. (n.d.-b). The whole body is involved in a golf swing. In *Unsplash*. https://unsplash.com/photos/kaZ6Uu54ZjE

Grebinets, T. (n.d.). A yoga mat makes exercising on the floor easier. In *Burst*. https://burst.shopify.com/photos/woman-preparing-for-yoga

Heath, C. (n.d.). Stability balls are great tools to strengthen the core. In *Unsplash*. https://unsplash.com/photos/xUCZbHydW-Y

Henry, M. (n.d.-a). A foam roller can ease knots out of hamstrings. In *Burst*. https://burst.shopify.com/photos/roller-product-used-on-hamstring?q=stretch+bands

Henry, M. (n.d.-b). Leg exercise with resistance bands. In *Burst*. https://burst.shopify.com/photos/tensor-band-lifestyle?q=stretch+bands

Henry, M. (n.d.-c). Resistance band leg stretch. In *Burst*. https://burst.shopify.com/photos/resistance-band-leg-stretch?q=resistance+bands+workout

Henry, M. (n.d.-d). Tensor squat band. In *Burst*. https://burst.shopify.com/photos/tensor-band-squats?q=loop+resistance+bands

LeJune, M. (n.d.). TRX resistance bands. In *Unsplash*. https://unsplash.com/photos/uU5Jz-b-0yI

Mars, B. (n.d.). Women with resistance bands. In *Unsplash*. https://unsplash.com/photos/oLStrTTMz2s

Pflug, S. (n.d.). Women with flexible bands, ready to do a chest press. In *Burst*. https://burst.shopify.com/photos/woman-strong-band-exercise?q=resistance+bands+workout

Pieters, G. (n.d.). Exercising with resistance bands. In *Unsplash*. https://unsplash.com/photos/3RnkZpDqsEI

Primeau, N. (n.d.). A healthy vegetable salad. In *Unsplash*. https://unsplash.com/photos/-ftWfohtjNw

Shopify Partners. (n.d.-a). A small fitness ball. In *Burst*. https://burst.shopify.com/photos/fitness-ball?q=gym

Shopify Partners. (n.d.-b). Dumbbells. In *Burst*. https://burst.shopify.com/photos/dumbbells-and-gym-shoes?q=resistance+training

Shopify Partners. (n.d.-c). Tubular resistance band. In *Burst*. https://burst.shopify.com/photos/fitness-product-squat-band?q=tubular+resistance+bands

Sikkema, K. (n.d.). Resistance tubing. In *Unsplash*. https://unsplash.com/photos/rWBBDErPXcY

Van, D. (n.d.). Resistance bands. In *Unsplash*. https://unsplash.com/photos/Mzu7qcmP5tk

Book 2:

Bodyweight

Workouts

Introduction

Are you looking forward to staying in shape and building your muscles? This ultimate guide will teach you about home workouts you can do without using any gym equipment.

You will learn how to stay fit, be healthy, and eat properly.

This book is suitable for men and women, but I will focus more on men (aged between 20 to 50) who want to perform effective bodyweight exercises in the comfort of their homes. You will be able to learn how to do the right exercise and work for different muscle groups.

In our first chapter, you will learn why you need bodyweight and strength-training exercises. You will also learn the basics of nutrition and incorporate the right diet with the right type of activity to stay fit and healthy.

You will also learn how to develop your workout plan and choose the right type of exercise to develop a particular muscle group. You will also learn how to determine what works for you based on your fitness goals and level.

With your fitness goal in mind, you will also be able to determine the number of reps you should do for each set and how many sets per workout. This approach ensures you have a balanced workout plan that works your whole body.

In this beginner workout plan, you will learn about different exercises that target your arms, neck, shoulders, chest, core, lower back, thighs, and leg muscles. These types of exercises will strengthen your body, increase flexibility and make you more balanced and stable.

There are many health benefits from doing bodyweight workouts. Keep reading to learn more about body weight and the different types of workouts you can do to keep fit and improve your wellbeing.

1
Bodyweight & Strength-Training Workouts

ARE you looking forward to building your muscles and staying fit? There are equipment-free bodyweight workout routines you can use to build your muscle mass and strengthen your cardiovascular and nervous system. You don't need any gym equipment to work out.

You can do the workouts from anywhere, so there is no excuse. Being on the road or a vacation with no place to work out and no equipment to use is no longer justification for not working out. You can easily do the workouts in your sitting room, garage, and even in your office—no need to subscribe to any gym membership fee or buy expensive training equipment.

Bodyweight training can help you:

- To effectively lose weight

- To build strength and body endurance levels

- To reduce the risk of injuries on your joints, ligaments, and other body parts.

Bodyweight exercises

Bodyweight exercises, also known as calisthenics, are a form of strength-training activities that rely on your body weight to provide resistance to the movement. They are intended to increase your strength, fitness, endurance, speed, flexibility, and balance.

Some exercises, such as bending, pushing, squatting, twisting, and more, are great for bodyweight training. You need just a little space to do most of these exercises.

Although you'll need some equipment for a few of the following workouts, most of them do not need any equipment. For the exercises that require a piece of equipment, you can utilize a common item in your home.

Bodyweight exercises are more convenient and deliver positive results. However, if you're looking to build muscle mass, you need to do the right at-home exercises and do them in quick progression to make the muscles more explosive.

Why bodyweight exercises

1. Time efficient

If you want to improve your body composition and stay fit, you don't have to spend more than 2 hours exercising. Bodyweight training is highly effective even when done 30 minutes daily.

All you need is high-output exercises, such as plyometrics and strength training, with little breaks between the exercises. You can easily transition from one movement to the next with little rest.

Doing short and intense workouts can yield better results!

2. Cost-effective

Bodyweight training requires only your body and the working space the size of your yoga mat. You can begin your exercises right at home without spending anything.

Some of the low-budget equipment you may need to aid in your exercises are sneakers, a resistance band, and a skipping rope. Although, these are optional.

3. Increase your flexibility

Bodyweight exercises work on your whole body, thereby making your muscles more flexible and improving the health of your joints. A full range of motion ensures the free movement of your joints and reduces injuries related to workouts.

4. Highly scalable

Bodyweight movements are ideal for everyone. Whether you want to stay fit, are in sports, or are weight lifting, you need bodyweight training exercises. You can make modifications to your workouts by using sturdy objects in your home. For example, using your chair to do squats or burpees.

With time, you will be able to build your strength and improve your motions, and you will no longer need the support of the objects.

5. Combines cardio and strength training

Combining strength-based movements with bodyweight movements, such as push-ups, mountain climbers, and burpees, will keep your heart pumping, burn more calories, build muscles and boost your strength.

6. Increases your balance

Increasing resistance while doing exercises will result in increased balance. For example, mastering how to do an advanced single-leg squat leads to improved body awareness and control. Finding your balance during your workout exercises helps you remain flexible and more independent with time.

7. Safe

Bodyweight exercises are safe to do, regardless of the type of exercise, age, gender, and level of fitness. Simple bodyweight movements can be used for rehabilitation to reduce aches or joint pains.

Doing the exercises regularly will leave you with healthy joints and bones. You will also have a lean muscle mass.

8. Better results

Bodyweight exercises engage several joints and muscles in each movement. Exercises, such as push-ups and lunges, result in measurable results. These exercises are more effective and offer excellent athletic performance.

Bodyweight exercises are more convenient and have endless variability. You can decide to do light movements or go hard. You can easily adjust from doing high-intensity sessions to doing a recovery walk. So, with various types of exercises, you can achieve your fitness goal.

The level of customization of these types of exercises is what makes them more preferred. You can always get what you need and when you need it.

You can also incorporate strength training into your bodyweight workouts to improve your performance. Based on your goals, you can use these workouts to stay in shape and improve your health and well-being. Bodyweight and strength training is also suitable for athletes of all fitness levels.

Strength Training

Strength training involves physical exercises designed to improve your strength and endurance. When done correctly, strength training can improve your overall health and well-being. For example, it leads to increased bone density, muscle tendons, improves joint functions, reduces injury potential, and increases ligament strength.

You can use your body weight or tools, such as resistance bands, to build your strength, endurance, and muscle mass. Implementing strength-training exercises into your workout routine will improve your performance.

Within just a few weeks into the exercises, you will notice some changes in your body. The exercises are helping you burn calories and achieve weight loss goals.

Why strength training?

* **Strong bones**

Strength training enables you to increase your bone density and improve your overall stiffness to the connective tissue. It helps reduce the risk of injuries because it enables stabilization of your body upon impact with external forces

- **Improve your body image**

Those who do strength training report that they feel excellent about their bodies after completing the resistance-training program.

- **Reduces body fat and builds lean muscles**

Consistent training will increase muscle mass and the body's metabolic rate (the rate at which the body burns calories while resting). The higher the metabolic rate, the more your body burns calories and maintains the other functions of the body.

The body burns calories during and after resistance training.

When doing strength training, you should follow a proper nutrition plan to see measurable results.

- **Help develop a better body mechanism**

Strength training can boost your body balance, coordination and improve your posture. If you always find yourself falling now and then, you can include strength training in your exercise routine to improve your body's balance.

Your balance depends on your muscle strength to keep you on your feet. The stronger the muscle, the more balance you have.

- **Help manage chronic diseases**

Strength training has various health benefits for individuals, especially those with chronic diseases, such as diabetes. Together, the exercises, along with the right nutrition, help them control and manage their conditions. For example, strength training helps reduce arthritis pain.

- **Improves your mood and boosts your energy levels**

Strength training increases the production of endorphins that is responsible for improving your mood and energy levels. The exercises also have a positive impact on your brain functions and improve your sleep quality.

- **Improve cardiovascular health**

Strength training, together with aerobic exercises, helps lower the risk of heart disease, boost your blood pressure, and reduces hypertension.

Principles of strength training

To obtain the best out of your training, you need to focus on these four fundamental principles:

1. Specificity

The principle of specificity states that the stresses you apply to your body while training should be the same as that of your favorite adventure. For example, if you have limited time to train, you should focus your time on the specific disciplines you want to do, such as walking or cycling.

So, if walking and cycling are part of your training routine, you should focus on them only.

2. Individualism

Everyone is different, and our bodies react differently to varying types of training exercises in different ways. So, if a specific type of exercise doesn't work for you like it's working for your friend, don't worry about yourself. Someone can get better results faster than the other while doing the same amount of training.

Some factors, such as pressure at work or home, can affect your training and overall results. Therefore, doing some exercise with your friend doesn't guarantee you the same results.

3. Progression

When starting, you can use simple steps to work out your muscles. As your body gets used to them, you can increase your workload and the resistance you put your body through.

Therefore, progression involves small increments. For example, increasing the stress you put your body through. Stress consists of the frequency of the workout, the duration, and the intensity of the workout. For example, you can start with a 30-minute walk today, the next day, you do a 45-minute walk until you can take a 5-hour walk every couple of days.

4. Overload

If you don't have enough rest in between the training, that may result in overtraining. You shouldn't confuse this with overload, where you increase the workload and implement the right amount of rest after each session.

If you properly increase your workload training and the right rest, it will result in overload. So if you're looking forward to improving your performance, you can employ the overload technique and avoid overtraining.

Bodyweight training tips for beginners

1. Make the best use of your warmup time

Before you begin your actual exercises, you can start up with a light warmup to prepare your body for the set of exercises. Doing a warmup will give you better results!

You can maximize your pre-workout time by doing stretches and 5 to 10 minutes of light cardio to boost your heart rate, as well as lubricate your joints.

2. Start with short and straightforward exercises

Start with a simple exercise that feels manageable to you. As you begin to build your strength, you can increase your workout intensity. If you started with five squats a day, you could keep increasing the number of squats every time you're exercising.

3. Avoid training to exhaustion

Do not overwork yourself if you feel you can't complete a set of workouts. You can end it before you completely exhaust yourself.

Chapter Summary

Bodyweight and strength training are essential for men who want to stay fit and build muscles. You don't have to go to the gym or use expensive equipment to achieve your workout goals.

Bodyweight workouts are also effective and efficient in building your muscle, increasing strength, endurance, flexibility, and creating balance. They also reduce the risk of injury and repair your body from the stress that comes with lifting heavyweights.

In the next chapter, you will learn how to get started with bodyweight workouts.

2
How To Get Started

STAYING in shape and having a healthy lifestyle is crucial. Doing regular exercises will help you achieve your desired results. However, doing the right exercises for your daily routine can be very overwhelming, especially if you're starting out or for those who exercise only a few times a week.

Further, incorporating workout exercises into your daily routine requires a lot of determination. You need the discipline to stick to your workout routine.

Getting started on your bodyweight-training journey will result in improved health and wellbeing. Exercise improves your mental ability, supports your weight-loss journey, and reduces the risk of chronic diseases.

Before you start any workout, you should:

1. Check your health

Consult your doctor or get a medical examination report before starting any workout routine to avoid any risk of injury during exercises.

2. Create a workout plan

Once you make your decision to do regular exercise, you need to come up with a plan that includes attainable steps and your training goals. You can start with some of the easy steps to do and continue building on it based on your fitness level.

Use progressive training principles to achieve your goals; starting with simple steps and carrying them to completion will determine your success. Doing a simple program will help you build a strong foundation and progress from one week to the next.

Achieving smaller milestones motivates and increases your chance of success.

3. Make it a habit

Once you start your workout routine, stick to it, and be consistent. If you make your workout exercises a habit, you will easily maintain your workout routine for the long term.

For example, you can develop a simple workout routine that works all your muscle groups three or more days a week.

Schedule a daily routine of exercises either in the morning or after work and make it a habit of following it.

4. Warm up first

Before you begin your exercises, you need to warm up your body first. Doing a warmup helps reduce the chances of injury when you start your workouts.

You can schedule 5 to 10 minutes of cardio or other warmup exercises.

5. Aim to challenge yourself

When starting, concentrate on doing each set of exercises rather than how many exercises you're doing. You will have enough time to improve your strength and build muscle mass.

How much exercise should you do?

You don't need to be an active or high-performance athlete for you to do daily exercises. You can start by doing 30 minutes of exercise a day.

The American College of Sports Medicine recommends 150 minutes of physical activity per week. The 150 minutes of moderate exercise can be reconfigured to 30 minutes for 5 days in a week or 2 to 3 sessions in a week. So, instead of spreading the 150 minutes throughout the week, you can have 3 sessions of 50 minutes each in a week.

It is also advisable to start with simple exercises and increase the exercise's intensity as your fitness level goes up.

Though you can make the exercises part of your daily routine for better health, including some rest is also essential for your body. If you don't give your body enough time to recover from the exercises' stress, it can increase the risk of injuries. Muscle strains and fractures can be caused by overstraining your body.

Too many exercises can also make your immune system weak, increase fatigue, create a hormonal imbalance and increase the risk of infections.

Planning Your Training Program

Are you thinking of starting your fitness journey? Building your workout routine is the first step to achieving your fitness goals and maintaining a healthy lifestyle. Your workout routine should include the plans, schedules, and the type of exercises to do.

A good workout plan should help you lose weight, maintain balance, coordination, and reduce the risk of chronic diseases.

When designing your plan, you should consider your age, nutrition strategy, lifestyle, free time, and goals.

You can quickly build your training program in these 5 easy steps:

1. Determine your fitness level

To start with, you need to know how fit you are. This will act as a benchmark to compare your progress. Your flexibility, body composition, and muscle density determine your fitness level. You can keep the record for comparison purposes. You should also choose:

- Your heart rate before and immediately after walking a distance of 1 km.

- How long did it take you to walk for 1 km?

- How many modified squats or push-ups can you do at a time?

- What is your body mass index?

- What is your waist circumference?

2. Come up with your fitness program.

Come up with your bodyweight workout routine for each day. Factors to consider when designing your fitness program;

- **Fitness goals**: What are your fitness goals? Do you want to lose weight? Do you want to build muscle? Are you preparing for a sports activity? Stating your goal will help you to stay focused and help you determine your progress.

- **What exercises to do**: Based on your goals, you need to develop exercises that will enable you to achieve the goal. What activities can help you lose weight or build muscles? Keep it simple. If you're a beginner, choose exercises you can do 2 to 3 days a week.

There are various muscle groups you can work on. If you're starting, you can choose one or two exercises to work your upper body and three or four exercises to work your lower body muscles.

You can select the type of exercise to do based on how your body feels. No matter the set of exercises you want to do, you should start with a 5-minute warmup with light cardio.

After the warmup, do a set of each exercise, one after the other, and take a 1-minute rest after each exercise session. After a while, with your routine exercises, you can modify them to be more intense. Always keep a note of how your body feels. This helps you keep track of your progress.

The workout routine you choose should have at least one exercise that works on the following muscles:

- Quads to work on your front leg muscles.

- Butt and hamstring exercises that work on muscles at the back of your legs.

- Push exercises to work on your chest, shoulders, and triceps.

- Pull exercises that work on your back and biceps.

- Core exercises for your lower back and abdomen.

Building a workout routine that focuses on 4 to 5 exercises can help you in working multiple muscles simultaneously.

- **A balanced routine**: You have created a balanced routine to help you achieve your goals. Department of Health and Human Services recommends that adults do moderate aerobic exercise for 150 minutes, intense aerobic exercises for 75 minutes, or a combination of the two. You should spread out exercises throughout the week.

The more exercises you do, the more the health benefits. Even being physically active for a short period during the day can contribute to your improved health.

You should include strength training exercises at least two times a week to work out major muscle groups. Do a single set of activities at a time focusing on your body weight as the resistance. Do at least 12 to 15 reps, which are enough to tire the muscles.

- **Start slow and progress slowly**: if you're a beginner, you should start with short and straightforward exercises and progress slowly. Ensure the fitness program can improve your motion range, strength, and endurance to avoid injuries. If you have any medical condition, you should consult with your doctor.

- **Incorporate exercises into your daily routine**: How much time can you slot for your workouts? Sometimes it may be challenging to get time to exercise, especially if you have a busy schedule. For your exercise program to work, you need to schedule a time for the exercises just like any other appointment. Your time commitment can help you design an efficient workout plan. Try building activity in your daily routine to make it easier to follow the plan. For example, you can take a break while at work to go for a walk.

- **Include different activities**: including various types of exercises keeps boredom at bay. You can include activities like swimming, biking that reduces injuries, or overworking some muscles or joints. Alternating from one activity to the other will ensure you work on all the muscles.

- **Include high-interval intensity exercises**: This involves doing high-intensity exercises for a short time followed by a recovery period of low-intensity exercises.

- **Include recovery time**: You should plan out the recovery period to allow your body to recover. Most people do exercises for days continuously without rest and only stop when they have injured joints or muscles.

- **Put it on paper**: Having a written plan will encourage you to stay on track.

3. Assemble the required tools

Always ensure you are in the right attire for your workout. If there are tools you need to use during your exercises, you can prepare them. To start with, make sure you have the right shoes based on the activity you want to do.

For example, cross-training sports shoes are great for giving the support you need during the exercises while running shoes are lighter.

You can buy a yoga mat for some types of exercises and a tracking device. If you want to keep track of distance covered, calories burned, and monitor your heart rate; you need a tracking device.

4. Get started

After creating your plan, you're ready to begin your training program. When starting your workouts, keep these tips in mind;

- **Start slowly and proceed gradually**: Always include enough time for warmup before beginning the exercises. Include gentle stretching to allow you to cool down. Then pick up your pace and proceed for about 5 to 10 minutes without getting overly tired.

When your stamina increases, you can increase your exercise time. Keep increasing until you can do 30 to 60 minutes of workout.

- **Break down the exercises if you have to**: You can schedule several sessions per day instead of doing all of them at once. Doing short exercises more frequently can be ideal for those with a busy schedule. You don't have to spend the whole 30 minutes doing exercises. Several short session exercises per day have aerobic benefits.

- **Be creative**: Don't be limited to the number of exercises you can do. Be more creative! For example, if you have been doing routine exercises such as bicycling, walking all week. You can include hiking with your family over the weekend and other activities. If you enjoy doing a particular activity, you can have it in your fitness routine.

- **Pay attention to your body**: You should listen more to your body, how do you feel after the exercises? Do you feel short of breath? Dizzy or nausea? Your body tells you a lot about your health. If you have been pushing yourself too much, it's time to take a break.

- **Be flexible**: If you don't feel well after a day of intense workout, take a break of a day or two for your body to recover before you resume the workouts.

5. Monitor your workout progress

After 3 to 4 weeks of your fitness program, you need to assess your progress. You can assess after every month to see whether you're on the right track to achieving your goal.

Sometimes you may notice you need to increase your exercise time to obtain measurable benefits.

If you didn't get the expected results, don't give up. You can set new goals and new activities to keep you motivated. You can also include your friend or family members to make the exercises more fun.

So creating your fitness program doesn't have to be hard. Proper planning and employing health habits will result in a healthy life and improved wellbeing.

How to determine workout days and rest days

To achieve your fitness goal, you need consistency. That is, you have to train regularly and over a long period. Therefore, you should create a program that is do-able and keeps you on top of the game.

The plan should have the right type of exercises and the rest. Come up with a simple schedule with all the activities to do throughout the week. This consists of 5 days of workout and 2 rest days.

The workout days should have a day of intense training followed by a recovery day with light exercises.

You should have 2 days for active recovery after intense exercises in the week. An active recovery day may involve doing exercises like going for a long walk, swimming, and Yoga.

How to determine the number of sets and reps to do

In every type of exercise you're going to do, you will come across the two keywords: rep and set. Rep (repetition) represents a single instance of a particular type of exercise, while a set represents the sequential number of repetitions performed—for example, 3 sets of 5 reps of push-ups.

A set involves completing a series of repetitive (reps) tasks that you do without stopping. For example, if you do 10 push-ups without stopping, you have done 1 set of 10 reps.

Choosing reps and sets sometimes can be challenging. However, your workout goals help determine how many sets and reps to do.

Rules to follow when setting up the reps:

- If you want to build muscles and burn fat simultaneously, the number of reps per set should be between 8 and 15.

- If you can do more than 15 reps with less difficulty, you can modify your activity to be more challenging.

Based on your goal, you can choose the number of reps you want to do per set.

- Doing reps in the range of between 1 and 5 help you build strength and super dense muscles

- Reps between 6 and 12 helps you build equal muscular strength and muscular size.

- While reps of above 12 help you increase your muscle endurance.

If you want to do high-intensity resistance, you can include 3 to 5 sets in your program. High-intensity resistance is excellent for men who want to improve strength within a short period instead of doing 8-10 reps.

When you're beginning your bodyweight program, you can start with few reps and increase the reps once you learn the movement.

Sample one week workout Plan

From the above steps, you can come up with your training program. The example below is an easy to follow workout plan for a week, and it doesn't need any equipment.

You can adjust it based on your fitness level and goal. You can modify it to be challenging as you want.

Monday: 40 minutes of doing a brisk walk or jogging at a moderate pace

Tuesday: Rest day

Wednesday: 10 minutes of brisk walk followed by the following set of exercises. Rest for 1 minute after completion of each set. Don't rest in between the exercises.

- 3 sets of 10 lunges on each leg, 10 push-ups, and 10 sit-ups.

- 3 sets of 10 air-squats, 10 chair-dips, and 10 jumping jacks.

Thursday: Active recovery day with Yoga

Friday: Bike ride for 30 minutes or go jogging at a moderate pace.

Saturday: Go for a 40-minute walk, run or jog

Sunday: Rest day

Chapter Summary

If you're planning to get in shape and build your muscles coming up with a training program will help you stay focused. A workout plan enables you to determine your fitness level and the goals you want to achieve.

Based on these two factors, you can come up with your schedule for the exercises to do. The plan will also help you determine what muscles to work out on each day and how long you should do the exercises.

You're also able to learn how to determine your workout days and the rest days and the number of sets and reps you have to do in each type of exercise. These factors will help you get started and ensure you achieve your fitness goals.

In the next chapter, you will learn how to strengthen your arms and triceps.

3

Five Best Strength-Training Warm-Up Exercises

BEFORE STARTING any form of workout, you need warm-up exercises to get your muscles started and ready for workouts that are more strenuous.

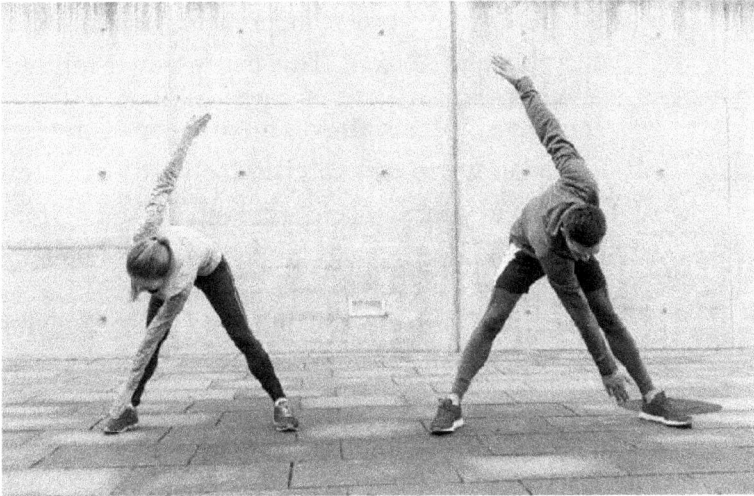

Sometimes, if you're short of time, you may be tempted to skip a warm-up section and jump-start your workouts. Doing this can result in muscle strain or increase the risk of injury. So, before starting any exercise, such as strength training, cardio workout, or sports, you must take 5 to 10 minutes to ease your muscles. The warm-ups help you achieve better results.

Benefits of doing warm-up exercises

Doing a warm-up exercise makes your workout sections much easier and prepares your muscle for strenuous activities. Some of the benefits of warm-up exercise include:

- **Increased flexibility**: This makes it easy to do the exercise moves correctly.

- **Lowers the risk of injury:** Doing a warm-up before any exercise can prepare your muscles and get them relaxed. This helps reduce injuries.

- **Increased blood flow and oxygen**: Stretches and other warm-up exercises increase blood flow and give your muscles the nourishment they need for an intense workout.

- **Have less muscle tension and pain**: Having relaxed muscles enables you to move them more easily. This will result in less pain and stiffness. You will also be able to drive your muscle joints easily.

- **Gain better performance**: Getting your muscles ready for the exercises increases the effectiveness of your workouts.

- **Increased heart rate**: The goal of a warm-up is to easily increase your heart rate to cope with the increased heart rate during workouts. Increased heart rate gets the blood flowing.

Dynamic Warm-up

You have probably heard of static stretching and dynamic warm-up and wondered what they mean.

A dynamic warm-up is a type of warm-up done to help start your workout routine. It prepares your body for more intense exercises. It focuses on making motions that are similar to the type of workouts you intend to do.

For example, you can do stretching movements that imitate movements, such as squats, lunges, or jogging.

Dynamic warm-ups help you build your mobility and improve your coordination. In return, this enhances the performance of your workouts.

Static Stretching

This is mostly done at the end of the exercises and helps calm your muscles after intense exercise.

Static stretching involves several stretches to help you lengthen or to loosen the muscles after intense exercise.

Stretches help improve your flexibility and boost your motions. Some of the stretches you can do include:

- Triceps stretches
- Hamstring stretch
- Hip flexor stretch
- Etc.

179

Warm-up exercises

1. Knee-to-chest stretch

Get into a standing position, then pull your right knee to your chest. You can use your hands to support your knees. Pull it as far as you can go and hold that position for 20 to 30 seconds. Lower your leg back down and repeat the same with your left knee.

This will stretch your hamstring and glute muscles in the back of your leg and increase your hip mobility.

You can also do this type of stretch while lying on your back.

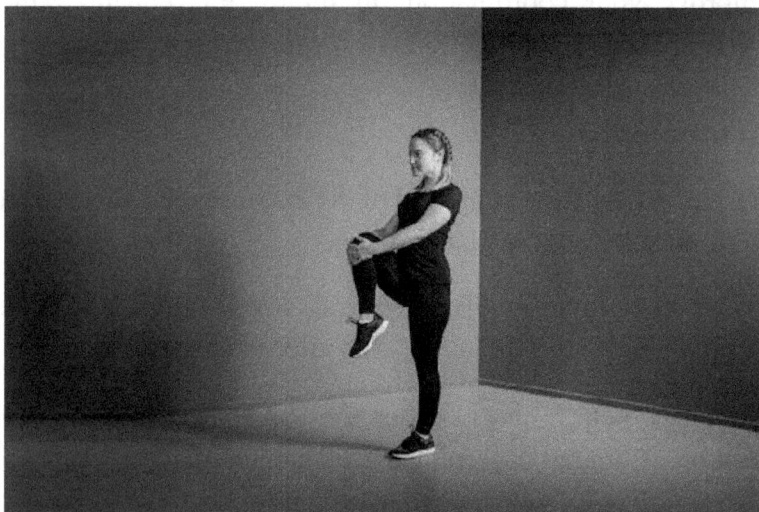

2. Quad Stretch

Get into a standing position, then lift your foot toward your back. Grab your foot while flexing your knee. Hold into that position for 20 to 30 seconds and repeat the same with the other leg.

The quad stretch works on your quadriceps muscles and hip flexors in the front of your leg.

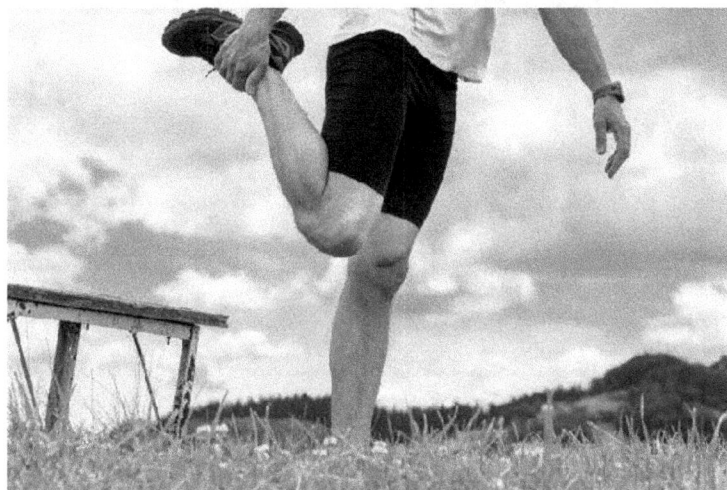

3. Triceps warm-up

This movement will help loosen up the triceps muscles. Get into a standing position and then extend your arms out to the sides. Keep your palms facing the floor.

Keep your arms straight, then start rotating them in a little forward circle for 20 seconds. Then rotate them in backward circles for another 20 seconds.

Extend your arms in front of you with palms facing upward. Then move your hand up and down for another 20 seconds.

Extend your left hand across your, then use the other hand to support yourself. Pull it as far as you can to feel the stretch and hold it in that position for 20 seconds, and repeat the same with the other hand.

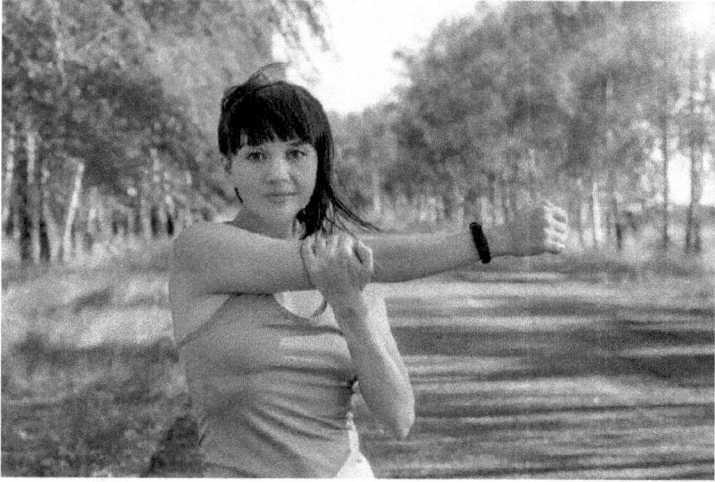

4. Jogging leg lifts

Doing jogging leg lifts keeps your heart pumping and increases blood circulation. It prepares your body for an intense workout.

Depending on the available space, you can jog in place or run back and forth if your area allows you. You can start with a walking pace by lifting your knees to your chest and increase your speed as you warm up. Do this for at least 30 seconds to one minute.

You can also kick your feet behind and toward your buttocks.

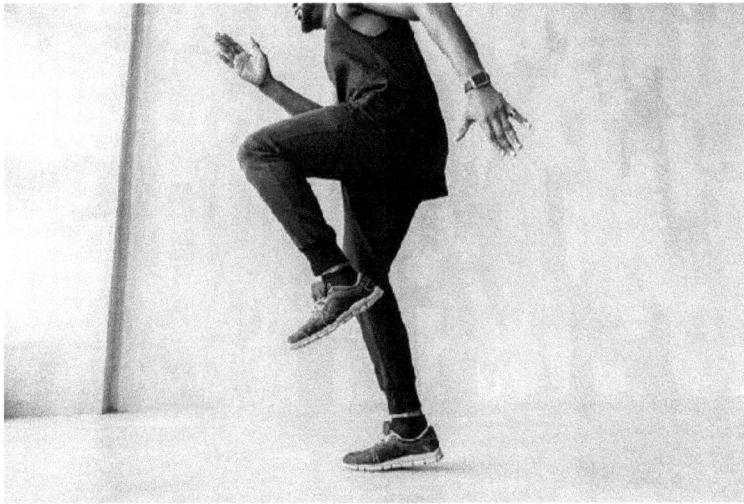

5. Side Lunges

This warm-up exercise works on your lower body and relaxes muscles on your legs, glute, and hips.

Get into a standing position with your feet at hip-width apart. Bend your left leg to be in 90 degrees and extend your right leg straight.

Hold into that position briefly, and then switch your legs. You can modify this by including squats. While your left knee is in a bent position and right leg straight, you can lower yourself into a squat position. Do this for eight to 15 reps and switch your legs to repeat the same on the other leg.

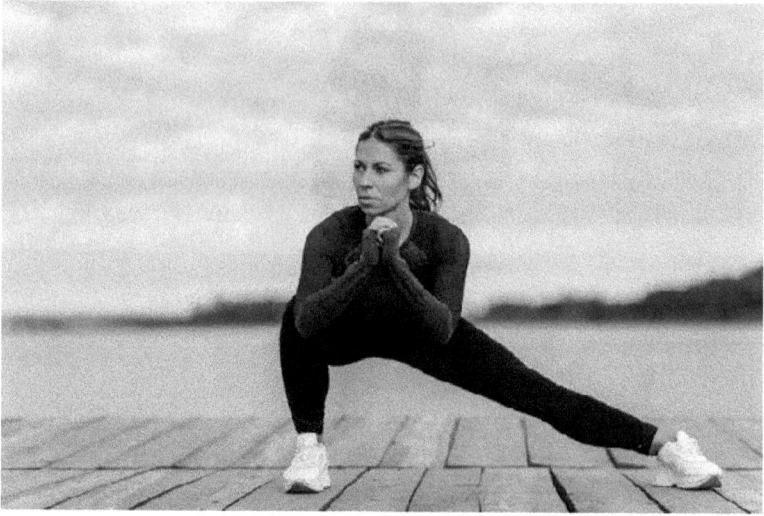

Chapter summary

Doing a warm-up exercise is essential because, during the strength-training exercises, the muscles shorten and lengthen. If the muscles are not well-prepped, they're prone to tearing and pulling, leading to some pain.

A warm-up not only activates your muscles but also helps increase your mobility and your body's core temperature. Different warm-ups work on different muscles on your body and loosen the tissue around your joints. This makes it easier to do the movements in your workout and increase your efficiency.

4

Bodyweight Exercises to Strengthen Arms

Do you want to have ripped arms? Your weight is enough to work on your upper body muscles—no need to lift those heavy weights to strengthen your arms. Bodyweight workouts are useful for working on your shoulders, biceps, and triceps.

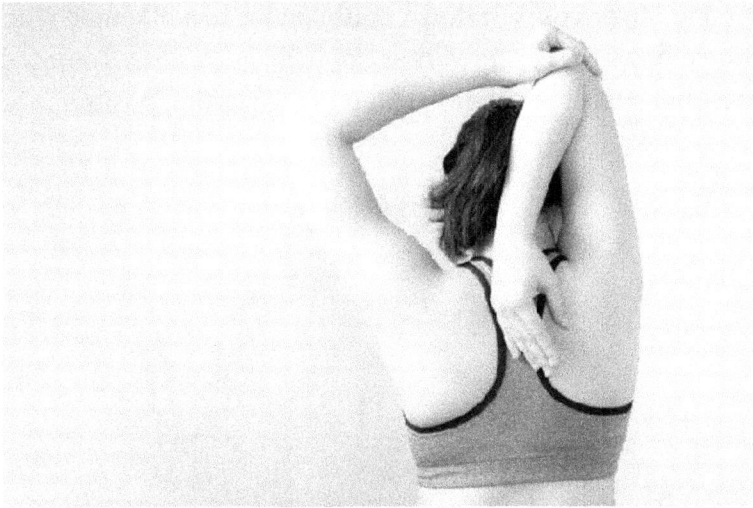

Most arm exercises with no equipment require you to use exercises that engage your core, such as planks and push-ups. This will allow you to work on both muscles at the same time.

No need for a gym subscription; you can work out those arms from anywhere. With a proper workout plan, you can quickly achieve your desired ripped arms.

The exercises require you to alter the position and angle of your body to make the right moves.

Bodyweight exercises for your arms

1. Dips

Dips are essential for building your triceps and forearms. They also strengthen your pecs and shoulders.

You can use a dip bar, a seat, or sofa at home to do this exercise. Facing away from the dip bar or seat, hold the dip bar and lower yourself down until you make a 90° angle with your elbows. When lowering yourself at the bar, keep the chest out. Raise yourself back up to the starting position.

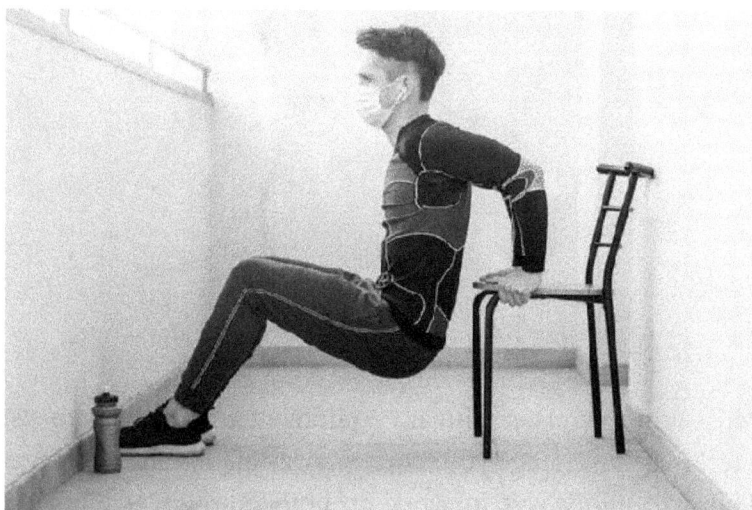

Ensure your neck and shoulders are relaxed. Walk your feet forward so that your butt is away from the chair's front edge and lower your hips towards the floor. You can keep the pressure off around your neck by looking at the ground in front of you, a few feet from you as you lower yourself.

You will find the exercise much more comfortable when your feet are close to the base of the chair.

Once you get the movement right, you can move your feet forward or lift one leg at a time as you make it more challenging.

To increase more strain around your pecs, you can bend your knees so that your feet are behind you.

If you want to focus on your triceps, you can extend your legs so that your toes point slightly in front of you.

2. Tricep dips with the lifted leg

Sit at the edge of a bench and place your hands on your hips so that the fingers point towards your feet.

Lift your butt off the bench and bend your legs to form a 90° angle.

Lift one leg straight and stretch it in front of you. Bend your elbow to an angle of 90°.

Push your back up to make sure your arms remain straight and repeat the step with the other leg.

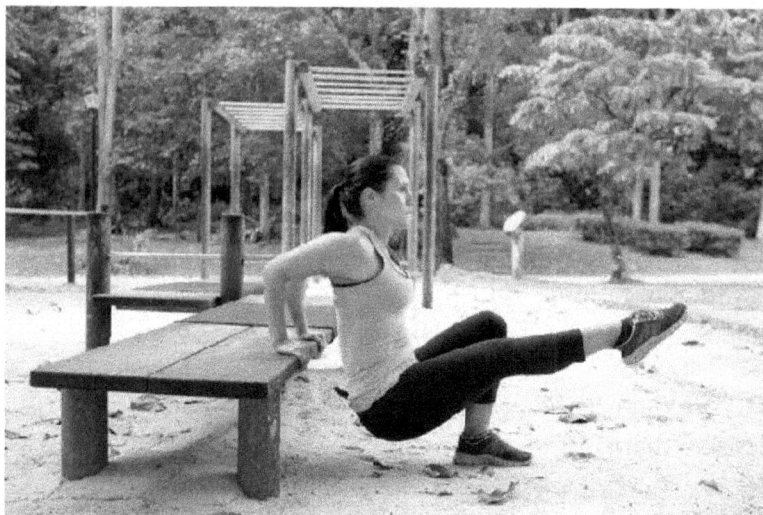

3. Pull-ups

Pull-ups are an effective exercise for strengthening your arms, shoulders, and back muscles. In this type of activity, you use your hands to suspend your body and pull up. It is one of the most challenging bodyweight exercises, and once you perfect the move, you can quickly build bigger arms.

Leap up and grab the bar with your hands. Firmly grip the bar with your palms facing away and shoulder-width apart.

Hang on the bar with your hands fully extended. If your feet are still on the ground, you can bend your legs around the knee. Keep your core engaged and your shoulders back.

Slowly pull your body up until your chin is above the bar, then slowly lower yourself down until your arms are extended again.

Aim to do six to 10 pull-ups.

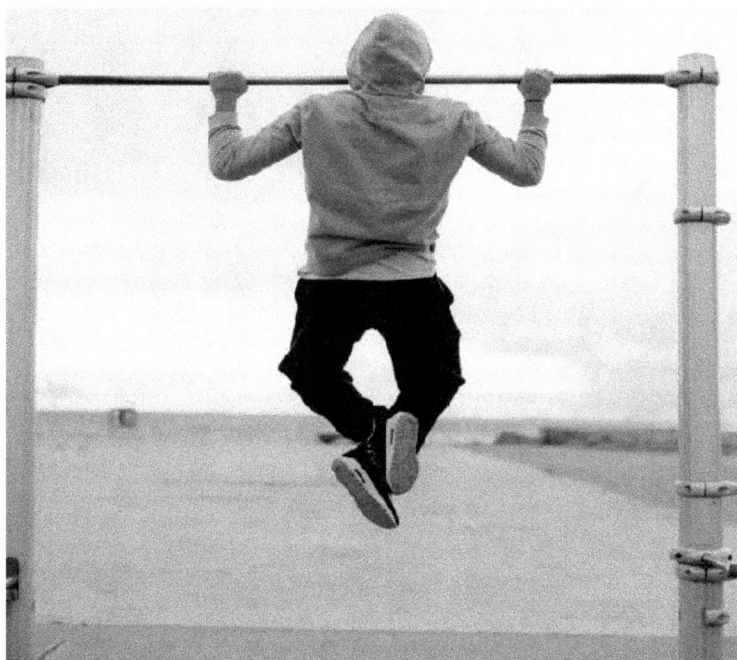

4. Chin-ups

A classic chin-up is similar to a pull-up exercise and even better working on your arms muscles than the pull-up. In chin-up, the palms are facing you! As a result, more workload is shifted to your biceps.

Just like in the pull-up exercise, grab the bar with your palms facing you. Extend your legs forward and your toes pointed, and then pull yourself up until your chin is above the bar. Slowly lower yourself down and repeat the movement.

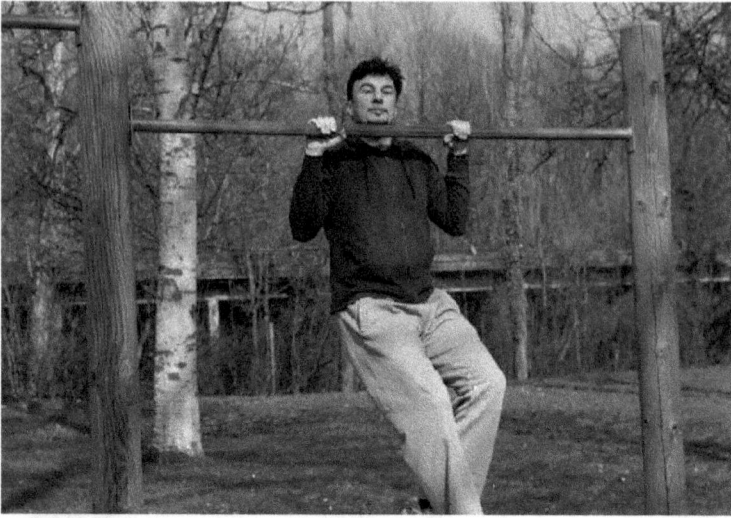

5. Plank

Plank is a core-strengthening exercise, and it is similar to push-up exercises. You should maintain a position similar to a push-up for as long as you can in a plank.

It works on several muscles simultaneously and is one of the best exercises for burning calories.

On your exercise mat, get into a push-up position with the toes and forearms facing forward on the floor. Your elbows should be underneath your shoulders, and bend them on the floor to form 90°. Lift your knees, and keep your torso straight so that your weight rests on your forearms.

Keep your head relaxed, and you should be looking on the floor as you maintain your body in a straight line (that is, from ears to your toes) with no bending.

The plank not only works on your arms and shoulders but also engages your abdominal muscles, as well, thus, drawing your navel toward the spine.

Hold this position for about 10 seconds. Do not arch your back or tilt your neck. The neck should be in line with your body.

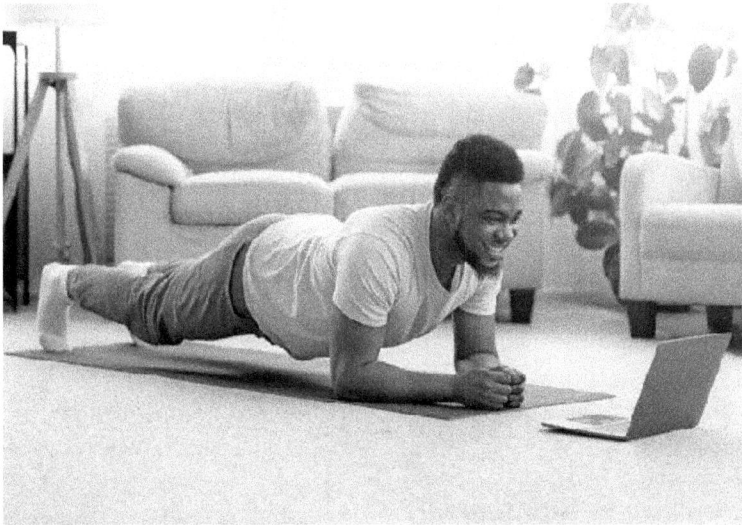

6. Up-and-down plank

This movement strengthens your shoulders, arms, core, glutes, and wrists. It helps in improving your posture and tightens your stomach.

Place your hands on the floor beneath your shoulders. Bend one arm such that your elbow and forearm are on the floor. Do the same to the other arm to form a forearm plank. Your elbows should be beneath the shoulders and alternative the hands to form a complete rep for a forearm plank.

Begin with the arm you started to back it up to form a high plank and do the same to the other arm.

Keep your hips and core tight as you do the movement.

If you find this movement difficult for you, you can put your knees on the ground to make the movement much easier.

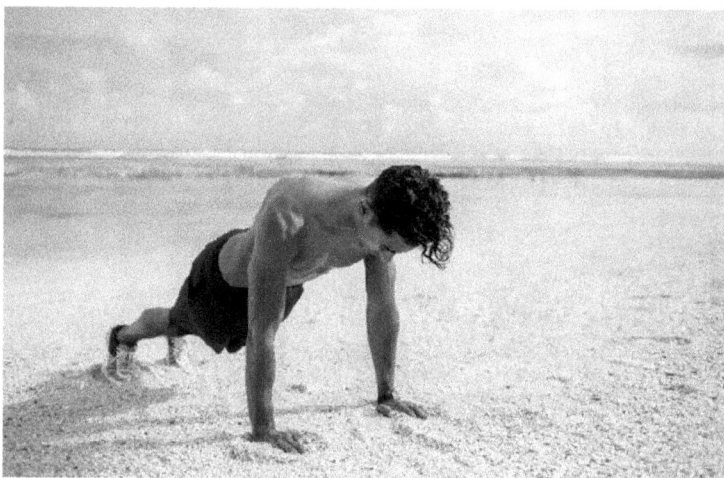

7. Inchworm with shoulder taps

Inchworm exercise works on your shoulders, arms, and your core. Start by standing, then form a forward fold by bending your waist and stretch your hands until you touch the floor in front of you. Walk your hands out to create a high plank position.

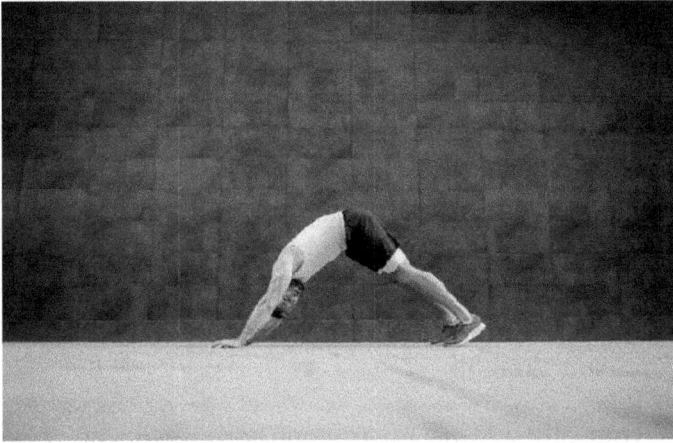

Walk your feet forward, one at a time, to meet the hands and complete your first rep.

You can bend your knees slightly to make it easier for you.

Lift your right hand and tap to the left shoulder. Do the same, on the other hand. When doing that, engage your core and glutes to keep your hips in position.

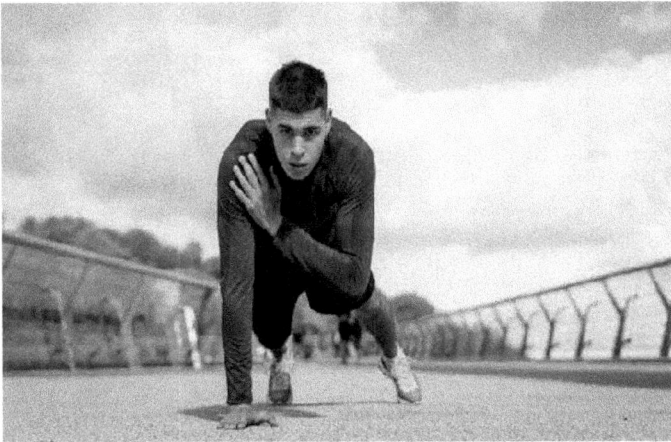

Walk your hands back in and go back to your standing position. Repeat the steps.

8. Push-ups

Push-ups help you tone your arm and chest muscles. Start by placing your knees on the floor. Put your hands on the floor and move your feet back to form the plank position. Adjust your hands to be directly beneath your shoulders.

Pull your body from your heels and position yourself a few inches from the floor. Engage your core muscles to help your body remain straight.

Bend your elbows and lower your body until you're a few inches from the floor. Straighten your elbows to go back to your starting position.

If you find this movement too hard for you, you can start by assuming a standing position then place your hands on a sturdy chair or against a wall.

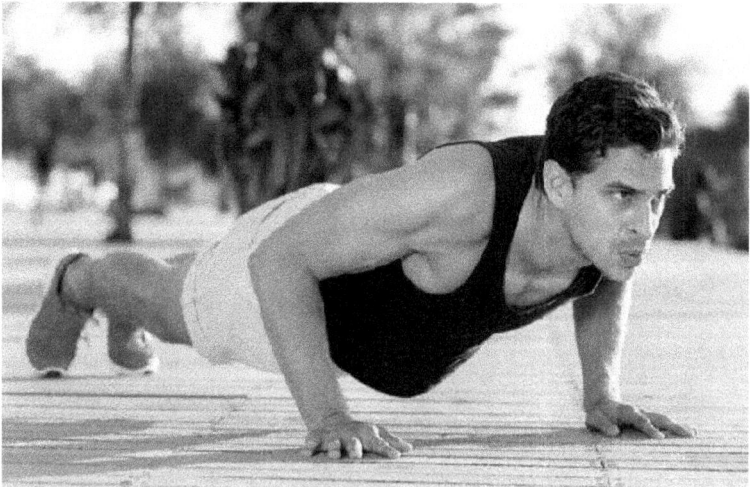

9. Triceps Push-ups

Get into a plank position with the hands underneath your chest and put your legs together. This will move the workload away from your chest to the back of your upper arms.

Position your hands such that your thumbs and index fingers form a triangle on the floor. Then, bend your elbows so that your body lowers a few inches toward the floor.

Hold on for a second, then extend your elbow back to the starting position. Ensure your core remains tight the entire time as you lower yourself toward the floor.

You can make this movement a little easier for you by dropping onto your knees and position your hips to be wide apart.

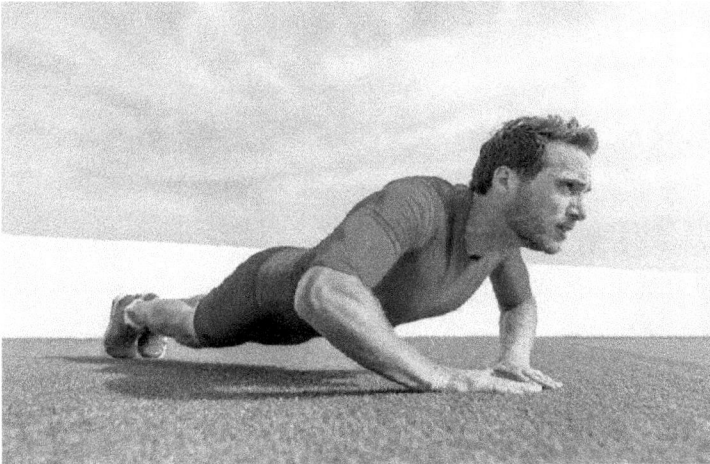

10. Elevated feet push-up

Elevated feet push-up is a modified bodyweight exercise that intensifies your movement. In this type of exercise, all your weight is shifted to your arms and chest.

This makes the exercise great for building your triceps strength and anterior deltoids. It also works on your pecs and core because you have to balance yourself so that the hips are not sagging.

It follows the same steps as a push-up exercise, but, in this case, you have to elevate your feet either on a bench or a sturdy box.

If you want to make the exercise a bit challenging, you can place your feet on a BOSU ball, which is slightly unstable.

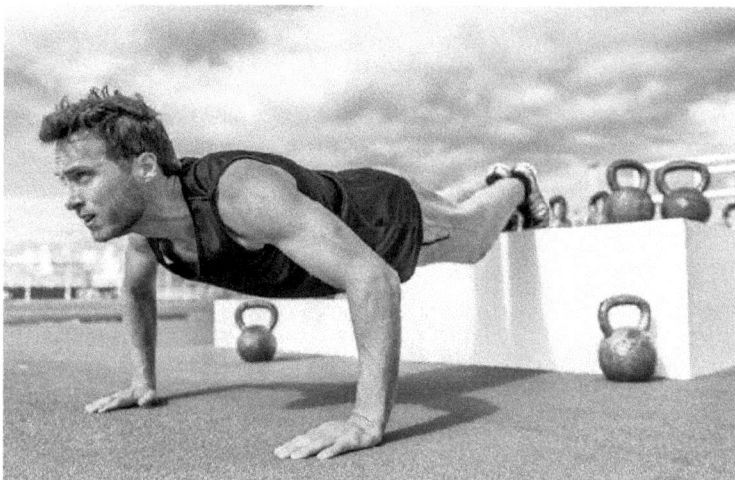

11. Pike Push-up

Though a pike push-up exercise is tough to achieve, it is perfect for working on your shoulders and triceps.

This type of exercise resembles overhead lifting where you face upside-down.

To do this, get into a push-up position and then raise the hips so that the upper body maintains a vertical position from the hands to the hips. You can easily get into this position if you place your feet on a bench.

This exercise requires you to learn how to balance your body and scale down the weight load on your shoulders.

Ensure your hips are maintained up the entire time, and your fingers should be pointing directly in front of you.

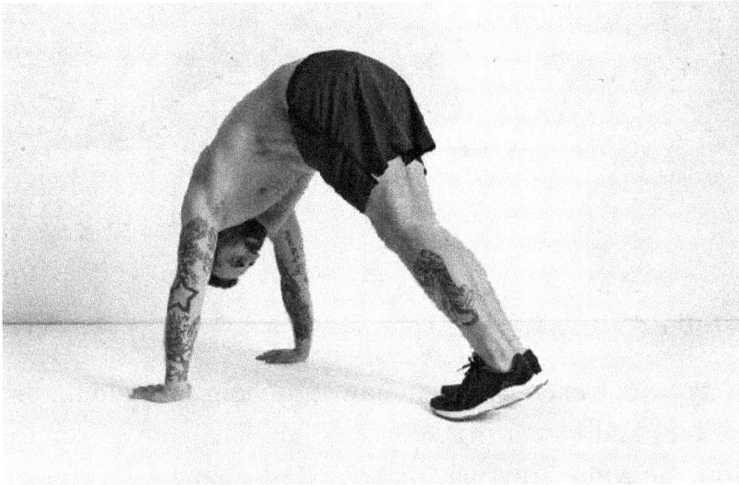

12. Crab crawl

Get into a sitting position on the floor or your yoga mat. Keep your palms and soles of your feet on the floor. Ensure your fingers are pointing onto your heels, then lift your hips slightly.

Move a step forward by moving your foot and the opposite hand at the same time. Move the other foot and hand simultaneously. Each step you move forward makes one rep.

If you find it hard to move forward in that position, you can lift your hips off the ground for about 5 to 10 seconds to complete a single rep.

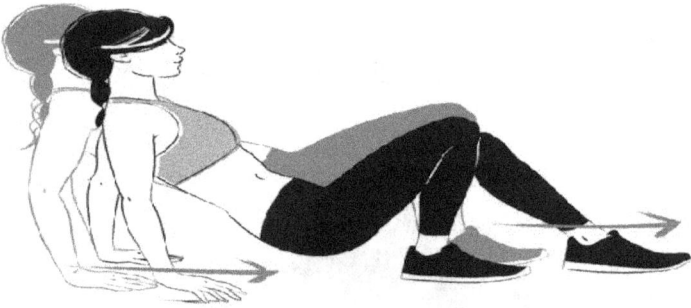

Chapter Summary

Bodyweight exercises for your arms help in building arm muscles and increasing your strength. The above exercises work on your arms and upper body to increase strength without using any equipment or weights.

Bodyweight exercises of building your arms muscles reduce the risk of injuries. Some of the activities also target your chest, shoulders and core muscles.

The workouts not only strengthen your muscles but also help you burn calories and boost your metabolism.

In the next chapter, you will learn how to work out your neck and shoulder muscles.

5
Neck and Shoulder Exercises

BOTH YOUR NECK and shoulders are extremely mobile, and a range of motions can leave them unstable and more susceptible to injuries. And, for those reasons, you need to strengthen them.

Shoulder and neck exercises offer several benefits. The exercises strengthen the supporting muscles around the shoulder joints and enhance your posture and stability.

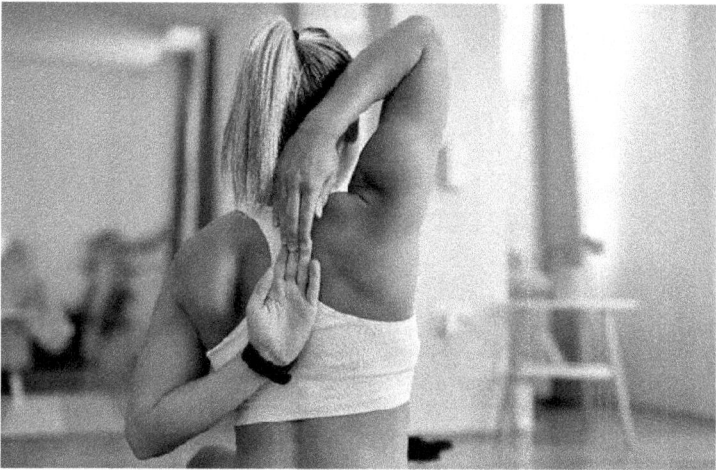

Strengthening your neck and shoulder muscles can improve your overall body structure. It also makes your shoulders strong enough to carry out your daily tasks without any injuries. There are also fewer chances of injuring yourself during the exercises.

Failure to work on these muscles can lead to impingement that limits your motion. The exercises make your shoulders more flexible and reduce stress on the shoulder joints.

Shoulder joints are very delicate because they're responsible for a range of movements. If you have weak muscles around your shoulder joints, your movement is affected, creating instability and injuries.

Therefore, the bodyweight exercises for your shoulders work on the rotator cuff (shoulder muscles) and the deltoid muscles. This helps prevent injuries!

Bodyweight exercises for your shoulders

These exercises allow you to tone your shoulder muscles while at the same time strengthening your ligaments and tendons. There are no weights required to do the exercises.

Shoulder exercises work on three types of muscles: Anterior deltoid, medial deltoid, and posterior deltoid. The anterior muscles are at the front, medial at the sides, while the posterior muscles are located on the rear (the back).

These exercises include:

1. Incline push-ups

Get into a plank position with your hands and shoulders elevated on a bench or box. Your upper body should be higher than your lower body. Lower your chest to a few inches above the bench, then push yourself back to the starting position, using your chest and triceps.

This technique works on your anterior deltoid and pectoral muscles. Your chest muscles are more active with incline push-ups compared to regular push-ups.

Ensure your shoulders and the feet are in a straight line, while at the same time your core and the hips remain engaged.

Doing three sets of 10 to 12 reps can give you better results within a short period.

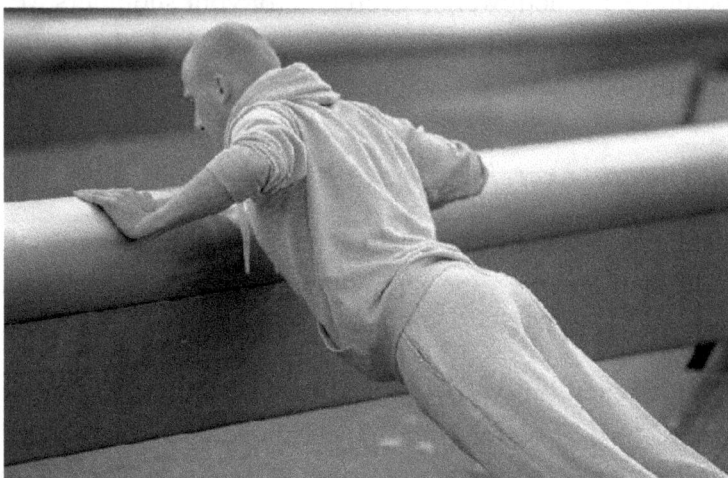

2. Push-back push-up

Get into a push-up position, then move your feet wider than shoulder-width. Lower yourself to the floor with your chest, then push your upper body toward your heels rather than push yourself up from the floor.

When you push the upper body toward your heels, go back to your starting position—this type of push-up works on your abdominal, deltoid, pectoral and tricep muscles.

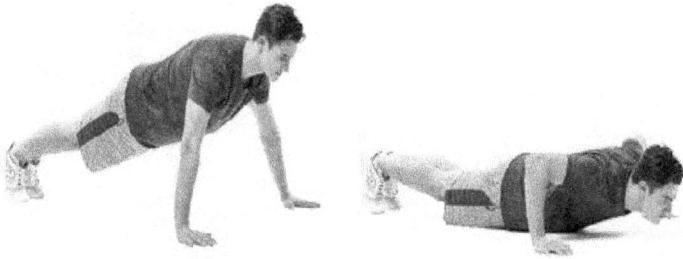

3. Plank to down dog

This type of exercise is excellent for working the rotator cuff. It increases your shoulder flexibility. Start by getting into a plank position with straight arms. Ensure your neck, shoulders, hips and ankles are in line.

Exhale, then lift your hips and move your head between your hands such that you create a straight line from your wrists to your hips and lower yourself back to the starting position.

Doing at least three sets of 20 reps can help you work on your biceps, hamstrings, shoulders and triceps.

Take your time to do the exercise; do not be quick when performing this exercise. Working on your hamstring muscles and calf flexibility will enable you to master the moves in this type of exercise.

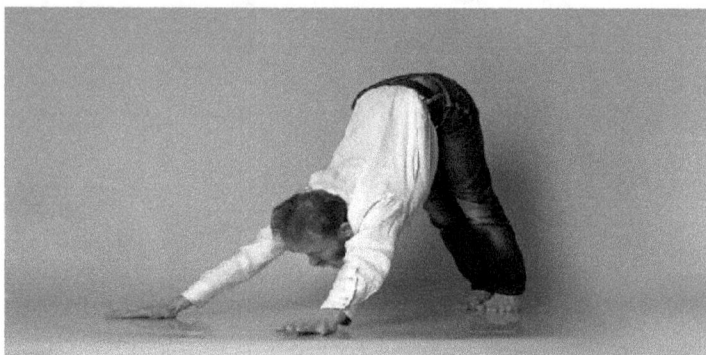

4. Elevated pike push-up

Like in a normal pike-push up, you can place your feet on a bench, chair or box and start the exercise. You can also get into a downward dog position with your elevated feet.

Keep your hands wider than your shoulder width, and the fingers should face forward.

Bend your elbows, then inhale, and at the same time slowly lower your head until it is an inch off the floor. While at it, your arms should form a goal post shape and keep a slight bend on your elbows.

Exhale as you push yourself back to the starting position and straighten your arms. Lowering yourself in this elevated pike push-up works on your shoulders and triceps.

To increase intensity on your shoulders, you should place your hands wider apart than the width of your shoulders. Do not lock your elbows, as this can put some load onto your joints.

PIKE PUSH-UPS

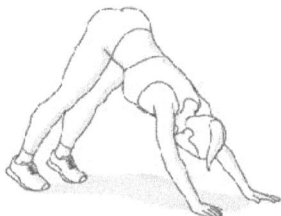
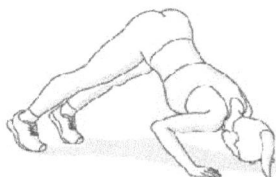

5. Plank-up

Get into plank position and put your elbows on the floor such that you form a straight line from your heels to your shoulders. Tighten your core, then start by placing the palm of one hand on the floor to push yourself up, followed by the other hand until you get into a push-up position.

Lower yourself back to the starting elbow plank position and repeat the movement one arm at a time. You can perform one rep when you're up with both arms and down with both arms. This type of exercise targets your triceps and abs.

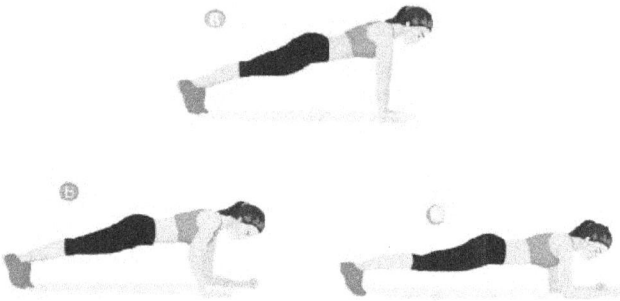

6. Wall walk

The wall walk is another bodyweight exercise you can do at home. It works on your abs, chest, back muscles and shoulders.

Get into a push-up position with your feet on the wall. Slowly back up and move your feet one at a time on the wall while moving your arms backward. Move until you're in a handstand position with your stomach a few inches towards the wall.

Slowly back down into the push-up position to complete one rep. Be slow when performing this type of exercise.

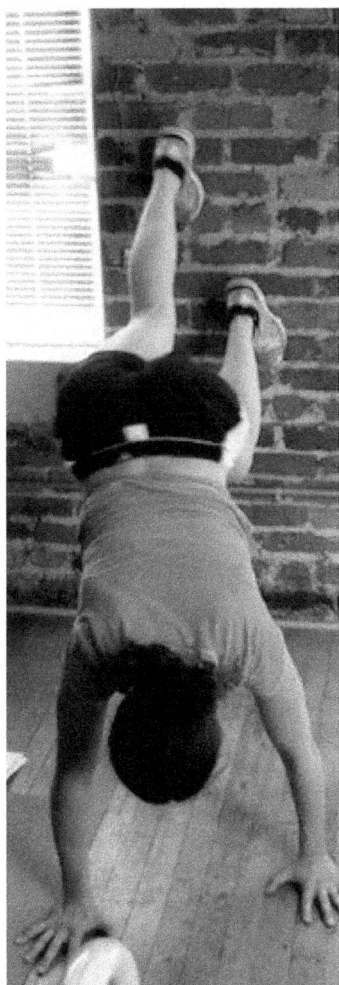

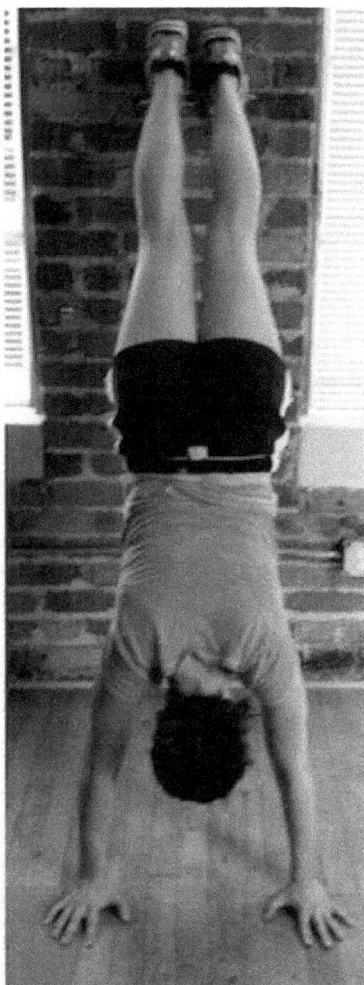

7. Crab walk

Sit on the floor and bend your knees. Your feet and shoulders should be wide apart and your palms behind you. Put your palms on the floor with fingers pointing forward.

Raise your hips off the floor and walk forward. Start by moving your left leg and right hand forward, followed by your right leg and left hand. Walk some steps, then use the same movement to walk back to your starting position.

This exercise requires you to engage your glutes and works your abdominal, glute, hamstring, tricep and quad muscles.

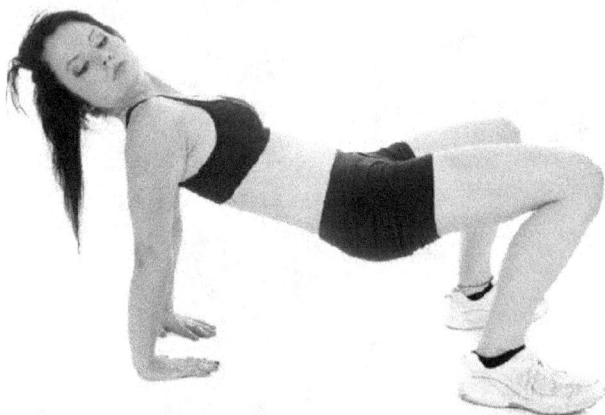

8. Reverse burpees

Stand on your feet wide apart (wider your shoulder width). Squat down, then lean forward with your arms out in your front. Put your arms on the floor like you want to do a push-up.

Get into a standard push-up position and ensure your body is in a straight line. Bend your elbows to lower your chest and body down to the ground.

Reverse your movement by pushing yourself up to the starting position. You can start up slowly until you get the correct moves, then speed up your movement.

You can advance your variation by jumping up after each rep and clap hands together over your head.

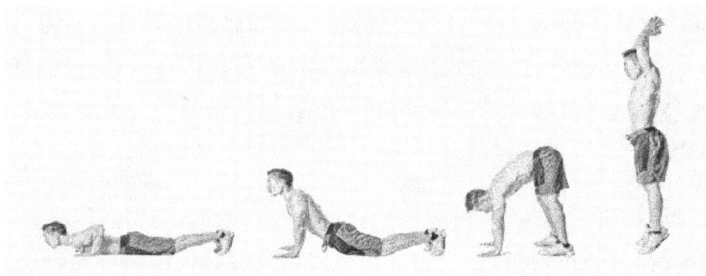

9. Handstand push-ups

The handstand push-up is an effective advanced workout for your shoulder muscles. You should be very careful when doing this type of exercise because a single mistake may result in an injury.

You can use a wall to support yourself and maintain the position as you perform the exercise.

Set a yoga mat or cushion against the wall, make yourself comfortable, and protect your head and neck.

Stand facing the wall, then put your hands on the floor with fingers spread to about 6 or 12 inches from the wall. Kick up until you get onto your hands. Place your heels on the wall for support.

Once you're inverted, straighten your body to be in a straight line and tighten your abs and, at the same time, squeeze your glutes.

Bend your elbows to enable you to lower yourself into the mat or cushion below your head. Control your body not to slam your head on the cushion or mat.

Once in the position, slowly extend your arms until you lock out your elbows to push your body back up. Do not rush with this type of exercise. Keep practicing until you're able to master the movement.

Handstand push-ups can be very difficult for a beginner, but with practice, you can get there. Before doing this exercise, you can start by getting into a reverse handstand position. And once you master how to kick-up into this reverse hand position, you can now advance to do handstand push-ups.

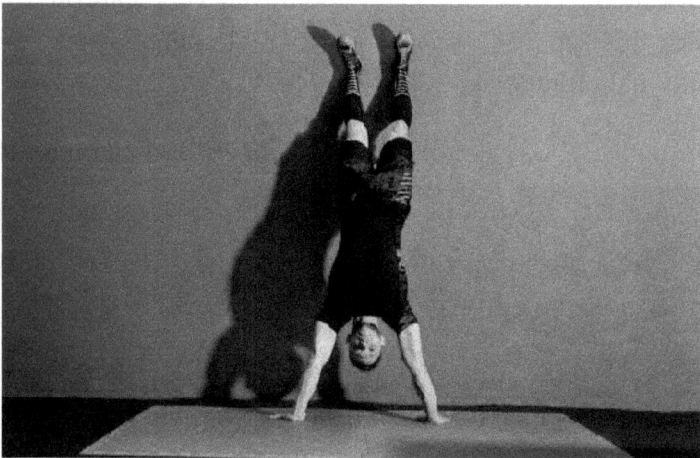

Neck-strengthening exercises

If you have a weak neck and upper back muscles, you tend to have a head that sags forward. It will also stress out the cervical spine resulting in increased neck pain. So, exercising your neck muscles will help you improve your posture and get your head into a neutral position.

Having strong neck muscles help reduce the levels of energy transmitted into the head during contact, and as a result, it prevents concussions.

The neck muscles include:

- Scalene muscle, found at the side of the neck

- Suboccipital muscle, found on the lower back of your head and at the top of the neck

- Postural muscles

- Upper thoracic extensors and deep cervical flexors

Most neck-strengthening exercises include:

1. Chin tuck

The chin tuck is the most effective neck-strengthening exercise that works on your postural muscles to combat any neck pain. This type of activity helps you strengthen neck muscles that pull your head back so that there is a proper alignment with the upper thoracic extensors' shoulders. At the same time, you will be able to stretch the scalene and suboccipital muscles.

To do this exercise, stand straight with your spine against a door jamb, pull your upper back, and head toward the door jamb. When pulling your head, ensure your chin and then pull the head until you touch the door jamb. Hold in that position for about five seconds and repeat the same 10 times.

When you pull your head and the upper back, you will feel some stretch on your scalene muscle that goes down to your collarbone. The scalene muscles, on the side of the neck, and the suboccipital muscle, found on the top of the neck, are very tight. Simultaneously, muscles at the front of your neck and upper back are very weak and require strengthening.

Once you have mastered the chin tuck exercise on a door jamb, you can easily do it while sitting or standing without any support of the door jamb.

You can do the exercise about five to seven times throughout the day.

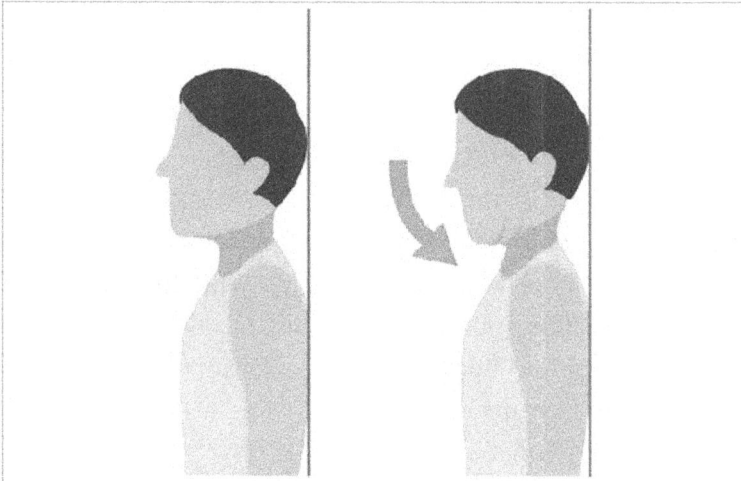

2. Prone cobra

Prone cobra is another strength-training workout that works on muscles around your neck, upper back and shoulder girdle.

To do this, lie on the floor with your face down. Place your forehead on a folded hand towel to make yourself more comfortable.

Place your arms on the sides with the palms touching the floor.

Move your shoulder blades toward each other and lift your hands off the floor. Move your elbows in, your palms out, and thumbs up.

Lift your forehead for about an inch off the hand towel with your eyes looking straight on the floor. Hold into that position for 10 seconds. Repeat the same 10 times.

Alternatively, you can raise your upper body with the arms on the floor and hold it in that position for 10 seconds.

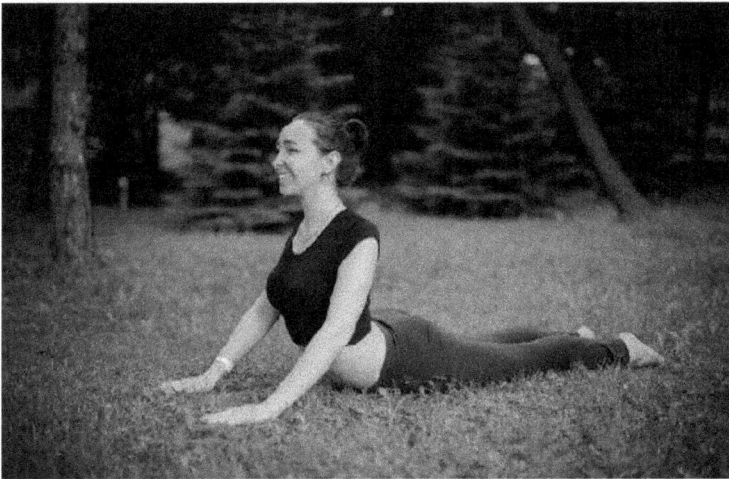

3. Back burn

The back burn exercise enables you to maintain your posture. Stand with your back against the wall with your feet four inches away from the wall. The back of your head should be touching the wall.

Flatten your lower back against the wall and extend your hands to touch the wall. The back of the hand together with your elbow, forearm and fingers should touch the wall. The wrists should be at the same height as your shoulders.

Slowly move your hands above the head and back down about 10 times. You can do this three to five times a day.

Doing daily exercises and stretches on your neck helps prevent any injuries and pain. These stretches can also be used to reduce pain in your neck.

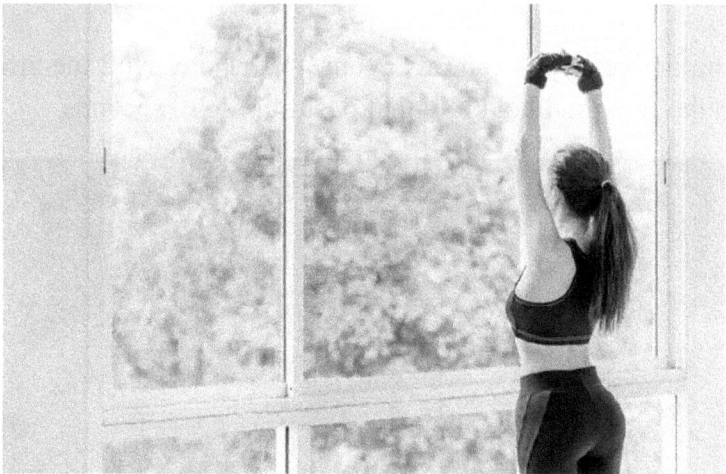

Stretches for neck and shoulders

1. Flexion stretch

Push your shoulders to your back, then bring your chin down toward your chest. Bend your head forward to make it easy to stretch the neck. When done correctly, you will feel a slight stretch at the back of your neck. Hold this position for about 15 to 30 seconds.

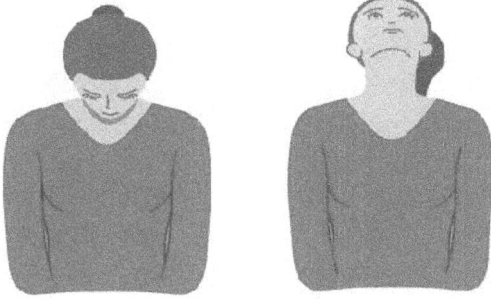

2. Lateral flexion stretch

To do this type of stretch, you need to be in your upright standing position and keep your shoulders even. Then bend your head to one side until your ear is toward the shoulder. You will feel a stretch on the side of your neck. Hold this position for 15 to 30 seconds and repeat the same process to the other side.

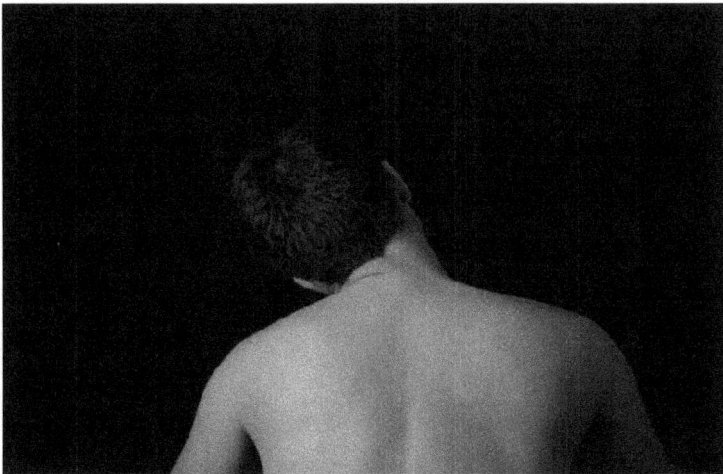

3. Corner stretch

Stand about two feet away from any corner in your house or doorway. Stand facing the corner with your feet together. Place your forearm on each of the wall or door jamb. Your elbows should be slightly below the height of your shoulders.

Lean forward until you feel a stretch on your chest and shoulders. If the stretch becomes uncomfortable, you can stop or reduce the stretch. Hold this position for about 30 to 60 seconds and repeat the same process three to five times.

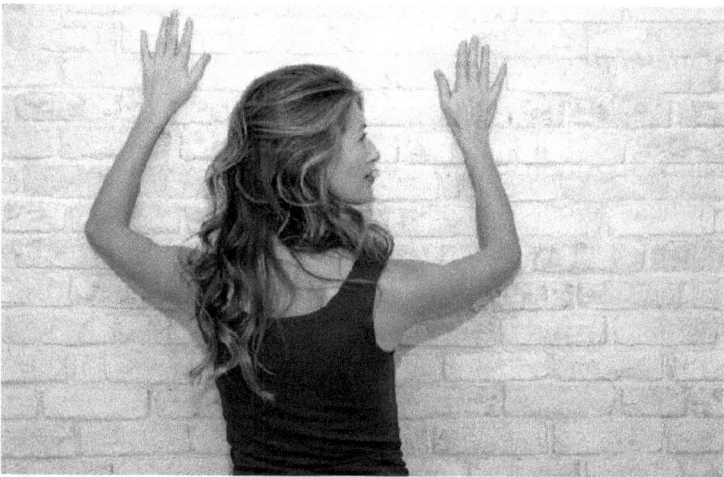

4. Levator scapula stretch

You need to stand straight in this type of stretch, lift your right hand and elbow and place them on the wall or a door jamb. Remain still, and move your head to an angle of 45° toward the left. This should rotate your head halfway toward the shoulder. Hold this position for about 30 to 60 seconds or as long as you can endure, then repeat the same stretch on the other side.

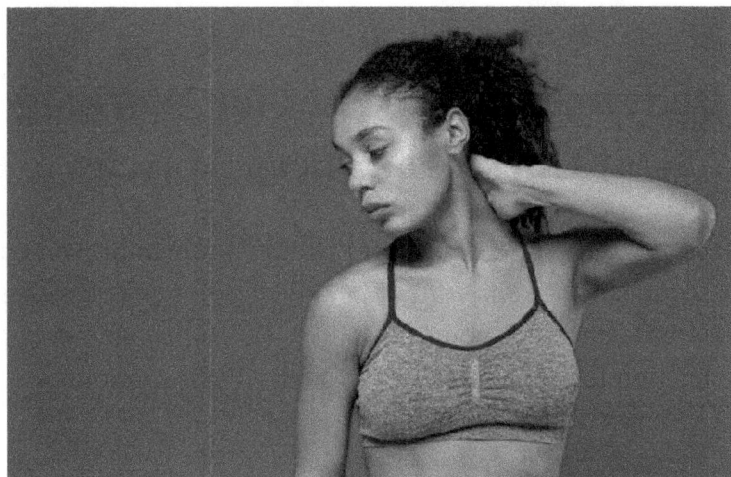

Chapter Summary

Neck and shoulder exercises are great for building and strengthening your neck muscles. The above exercises can help you in releasing the tension and stiffness. Shoulder and neck bodyweight workouts can also help you reduce pains and loosen muscle tightness, increasing your flexibility.

When starting the exercises, move at a slow pace and increase the intensity of the exercises and duration as you progress. Make your neck-stretching exercises part of your daily routine for better results.

Avoid overworking your neck and shoulder muscles, as this can result in injuries and pain. Do not stress or strain the muscles. If a particular exercise doesn't feel right for you, don't do it.

In the next chapter, you will learn bodyweight exercises for working out your chest muscles.

6
Bodyweight Exercises for Working Out Chest And Bicep Muscles

WORKING out your chest (pecs) will help you improve your physique and stabilize your shoulder joints. Your chest muscles support all your daily body functions and act as a foundation for doing a variety of bodyweight workouts.

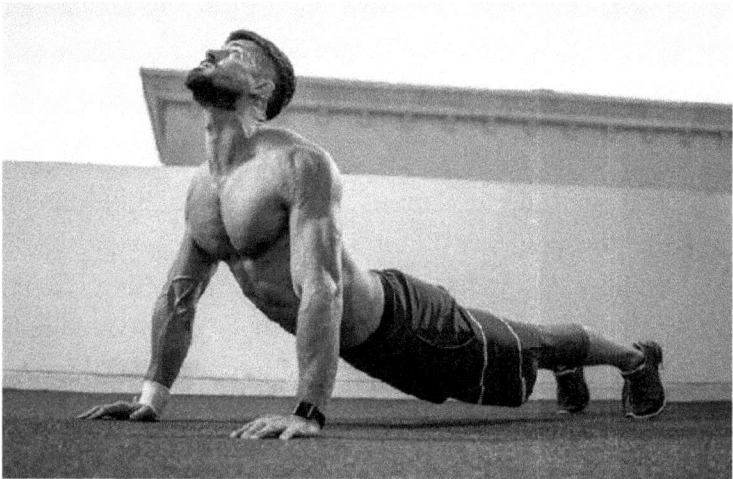

The pecs consist of the pectoralis major and pectoralis minor. Pectoralis major is the large muscle that forms most of the chest muscles. This muscle type consists of the clavicular head on the upper portion and a sternal head on the lower part.

Your chest muscles control the movement of your arms up, down and across. The muscles allow you to carry out your daily activities. Some exercises, such as push-ups, require the use of chest muscles. They also allow you to burn more calories since the muscles can handle more weight.

Chest muscles act as a warm-up on working out the smaller muscles. Different types of exercises strengthen your chest muscles and work on your arms and shoulder muscles. Chest muscles help improve your posture, lengthen your chest and support deep breathing.

In addition to working on your back and shoulder muscles, chest muscles help improve your breathing.

Exercises to build chest muscles

1. Traditional push-up

Push-ups are great for working on your chest and arms. You can do the push-up from anywhere and at any time. It needs only a firm surface and your body weight.

Push-ups work on several small muscle groups and requires you to engage your core and hip flexor muscles.

Place your hands on the floor and ensure they're shoulder-width apart. Brace your abs and keep your body in a straight line. Lower yourself down until you're a few inches off the floor and squeeze the shoulder blades together.

You can perform a wide push-up where your hands are placed wider apart than the standard shoulder-width for more variation. A wide push-up puts more pressure on your chest because more weight is transferred to your pectoral muscles. It will also help you strengthen your upper body.

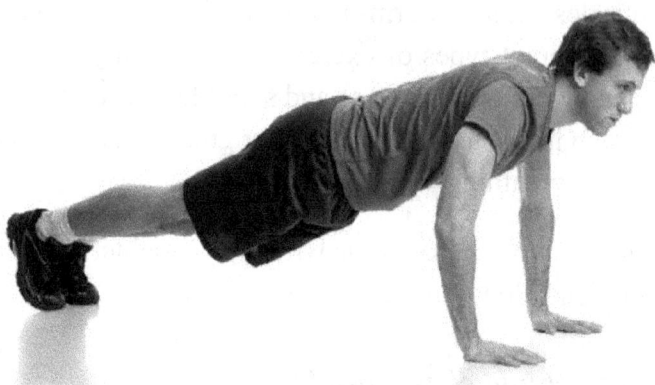

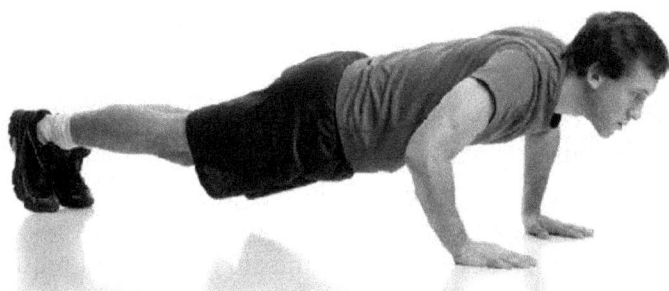

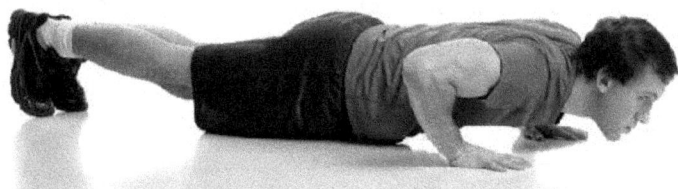

2. Decline push-ups

This is a variation of the traditional push-up. In this, you put your feet on a higher ground than your hands. For example, you can place your feet on a bench, a box, or a chair. The higher the level, the more intense the exercise gets. You may find it challenging to do initially, but once you master the movement, you'll be able to easily do them, and this will get you better results.

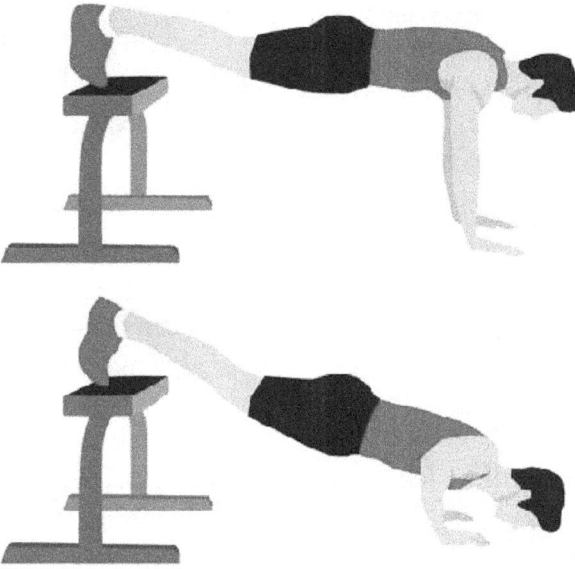

3. Diamond push-ups

Diamond push-ups are another variation for doing more intense exercises. Put your hands close together so that your thumb and index finger touch each other to form a diamond shape. Once your hands are in position, do the push-ups.

This movement will work on your triceps and the inner chest muscles. You can do seven to 10 reps to get better results.

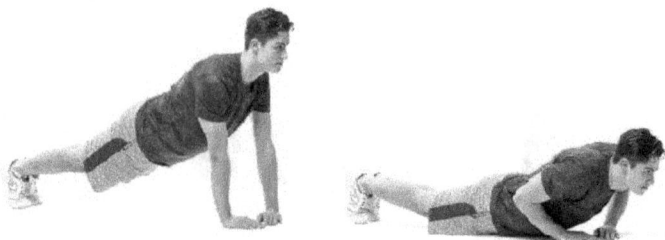

4. Push-up hold

A push-up hold is an isometric form of exercise strengthening your core, shoulder and arm muscles. It makes you strong—not only physically but also mentally.

In this type of workout, you hold your body up in the basic push-up position for as long as you can. Holding in the lowered position can be difficult for those who find it challenging to do the basic push-up position.

The push-up hold enables you to push your limits. The key to your success depends on your belief.

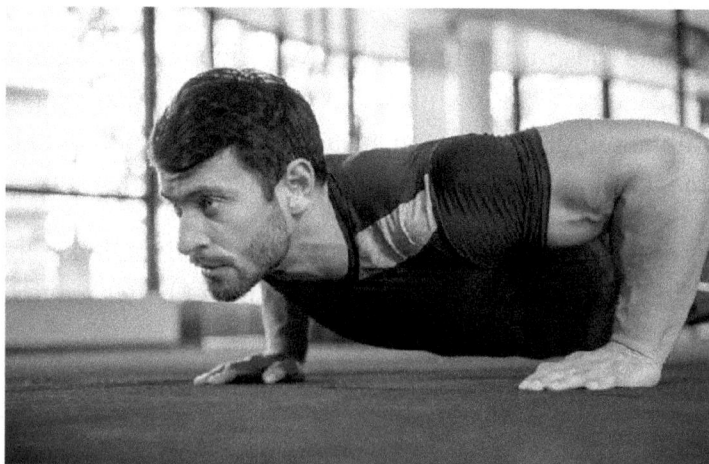

5. Dive-bomber push-up

Start by getting into a push-up position. Put your hands on the floor and raise your hips into the air. Keep your back straight and your head behind your hands.

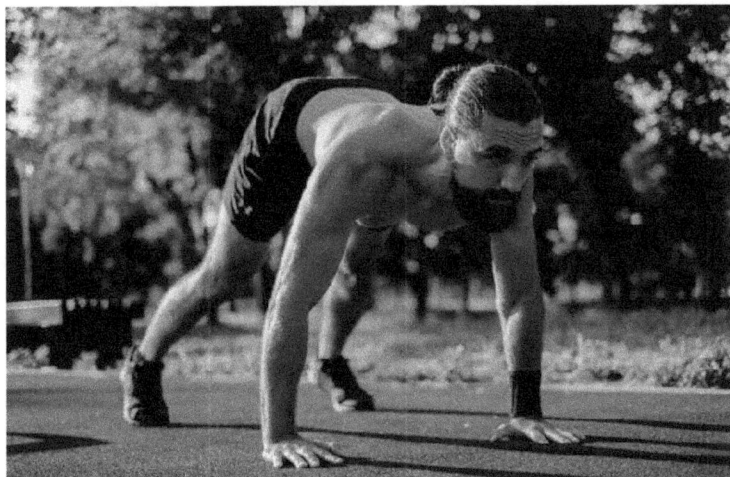

Lower your body to be in arcing motion and your chest a few inches off the floor. Push your body forward until your torso is vertical, while your legs are straight on the floor.

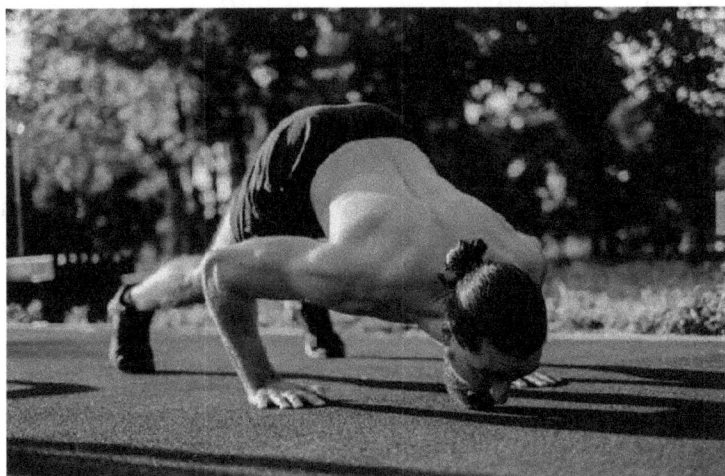

6. Star plank

Star plank movement works on your chest and arm muscles. Start by getting into a push-up position. Move your hands and feet to be wide apart such that your body makes a star shape.

Hold that position for as long as you can. Keep your torso straight and brace your abs.

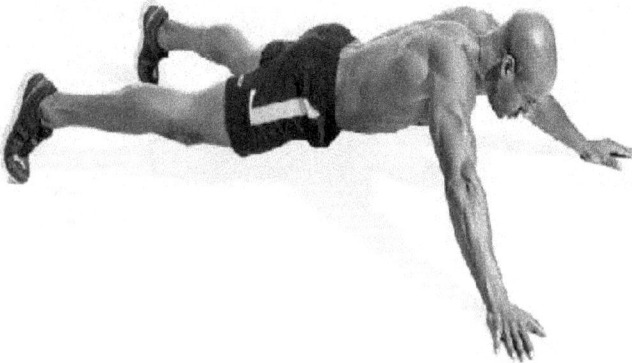

7. Plank reach under

Get into a plank position with your arms placed within shoulder-width (beneath your shoulders). While still in the plank position, lift your left arm and touch your right knee. Then get back to the plank position and repeat the same using the right arm.

Alternate your arms to do eight to 10 reps without any rest.

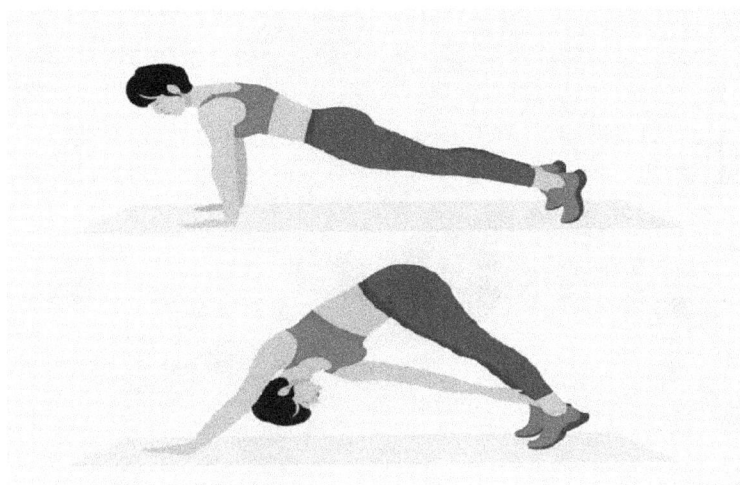

8. Side plank

In a side plank, you engage your shoulder and bicep muscles.

Start this movement with your right side. Place your right hand on the floor and extend your arm so that it forms a straight line from your ankles up to the shoulders.

Lift the left leg to ensure only the sides of your right foot and the palm of your right hand touch the floor. Hold that position for as long as you can.

Repeat the same step on your left side.

You can modify this movement by placing your forearm on the floor instead of the palms of your hand.

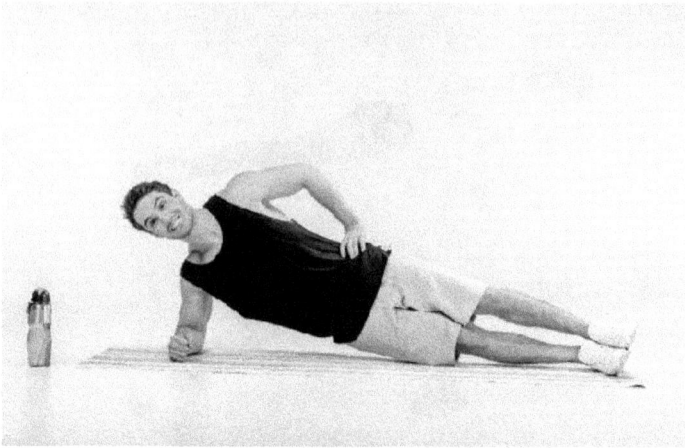

9. Chaturanga

Chaturanga is a classic yoga move, and you can use it to work on your biceps and core muscles.

Start by getting into a standard plank position with your hands on the floor and elbows beneath your shoulders at an angle of 90°. Lower yourself down to be a few inches off the floor. Push your elbows to be at the same height as your sides.

The move also helps work on your toe muscles. For better results, align your chest, elbows, upper arms and shoulders. Then push yourself back to the plank position and repeat the movement.

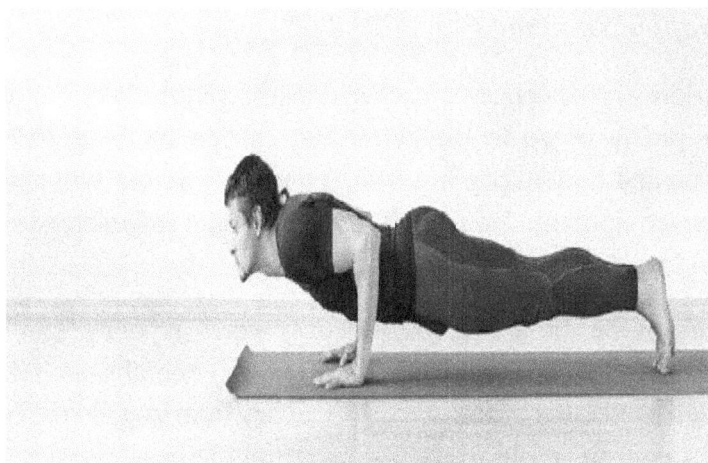

10. Resistance band biceps curl

Pick your resistance band or a towel and sit on the floor. Tuck your knees under you and straighten your spine.

Take your resistance band and slide it under your right knee. Grab it using your hand and pull it toward your right shoulder. Ensure your right arm stays in place.

Release the hold and repeat the same steps on your left knee.

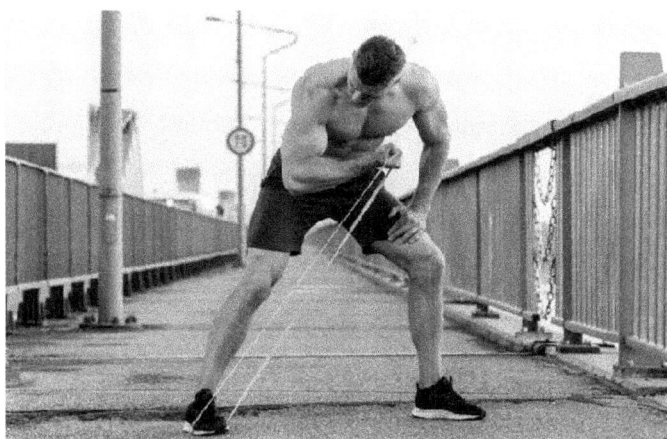

Chapter Summary

Building your chest muscles doesn't require you to use equipment or go to the gym. You can do the exercises at home and build a bigger chest. Your bodyweight will act as your equipment. You don't need complicated exercises to build your chest muscles.

Some of the above exercises not only work on your pectoralis major and minor, but they also target your abs, deltoids, triceps and other types of muscles. They help you get the best muscles you would want to show off at the beach.

In the next chapter, you will learn exercises you can use to build your core and back.

7

Bodyweight Exercises to Work on Your Core and Back Muscles

EXERCISING your core and back muscles helps you strengthen the key muscles that cause hunched shoulders and reduce back pain. Doing the right type of exercises increase your blood flow on your lower back and reduce stiffness.

Bodyweight exercises require high levels of core stability. To have a stable core, you need to work both abs and back muscles together. Otherwise, you will not get strong by merely focusing on a single muscle.

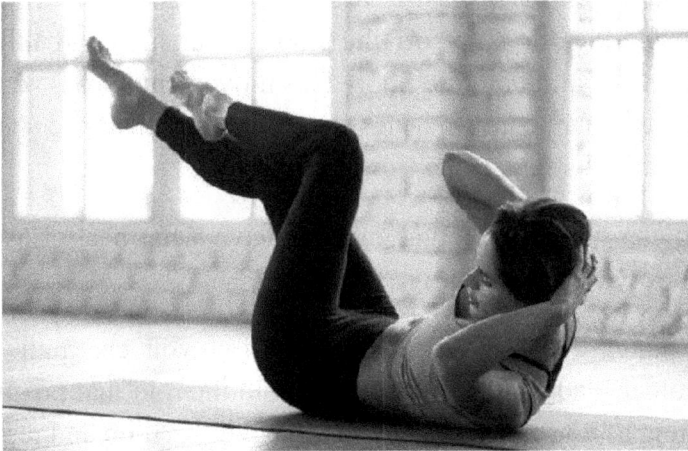

Your body weight is enough to work out your back and core muscles. Although some movements require you to pull up bars and straps but the only resistance you need to work against comes from your body weight.

You should also come up with a perfect workout plan for your back and core. And do a warm-up before you begin any exercise to activate your deep core muscles. A warm-up helps you get the best out of the exercises and also prevent injuries.

Simple exercises for your back and core muscles

1. Low plank

Lie on your stomach with your hands extended forward, then bend your elbows to be at 90° and place your forearms on the floor. Your elbows should be directly beneath your shoulders.

Extend your legs, ensure your toes touch the floor, and slowly lift your body off the floor. Your hips and thighs should be parallel to the floor. This movement allows you to engage your core muscles and ensures that the body maintains a straight line from head to feet.

You can tuck your pelvis under to have a flat back. Ensure your lower back doesn't sag or lift.

To increase the movement's intensity, you can pull the shoulder blades in and down and hold them in that position as long as you can. Get back to the plank position and repeat the movement.

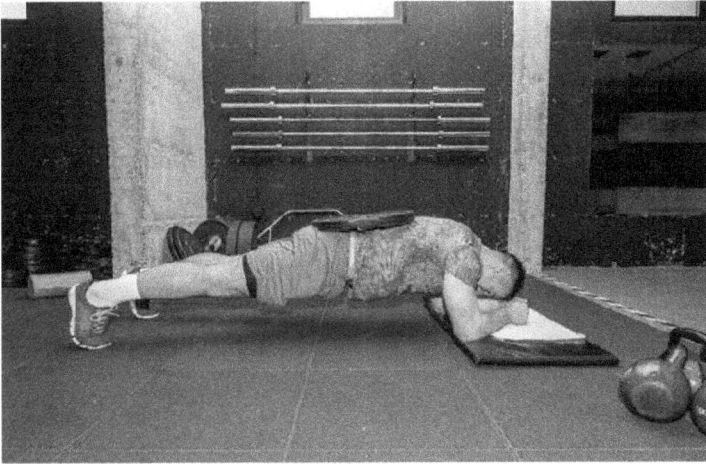

2. High plank

Get into a standard plank position with your hands placed shoulder-width apart on the floor and slightly bend your elbows.

Extend your legs and rest your toes on the floor.

Lift your hips and thighs to be diagonal to the floor. Engage the core muscles so that your body is straight from head to feet.

Tuck in your pelvis to form a flat back. Do not sag or lift your lower back or the lumbar region. Then pull your shoulder blades in and down and hold for as long as you can.

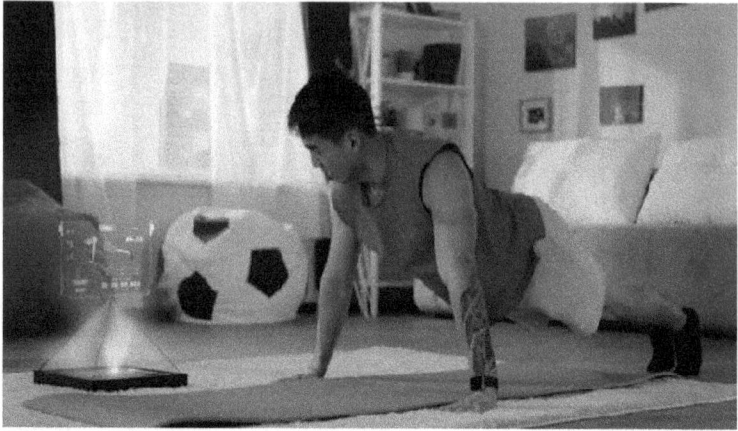

3. Bridge

You have to lie on your back with your face up and your head on the floor for this bridge exercise. Bend your knees so that your heels are directly beneath your knees. Keep your hands on your sides near your hips with your palms facing down to add balance.

Tuck your pelvis region to have a flat lower back, and then pull the shoulder blades in and down and hold them in that position. Lift your hips high until fully extended, then hold that position for about 10 seconds. Your knees, hips, and shoulders should be in a straight line. While on it, squeeze your glutes, then lower your hips back to a few inches off the floor.

Repeat the movement.

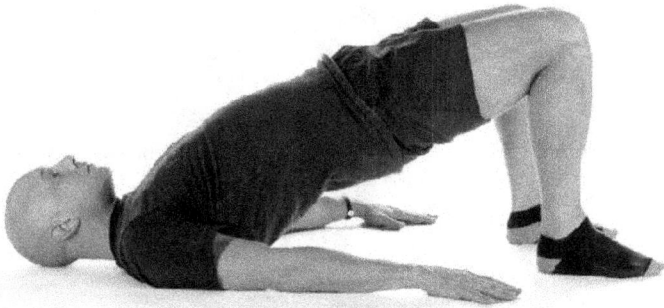

4. *Superman*

Superman is another bodyweight exercise that works on your upper and lower back, abs, core muscles, glutes and shoulders. Start by lying flat on your stomach with your hands stretched forward, palms placed on the floor.

Raise your legs and upper body off the floor to form an arch-like shape. Your knees and chest shouldn't touch the floor. Raise your head and tuck in your chin, and don't overextend your neck.

Extend your hands forward. You can also slightly bend the elbows as you extend them. You can increase the core tension by slightly raising the upper body and legs higher at the same time.

When doing the superman move, don't look up, as this can make you stretch your neck, making you feel uncomfortable. Make sure you lie on a yoga mat or carpet to ensure you're comfortable doing this exercise.

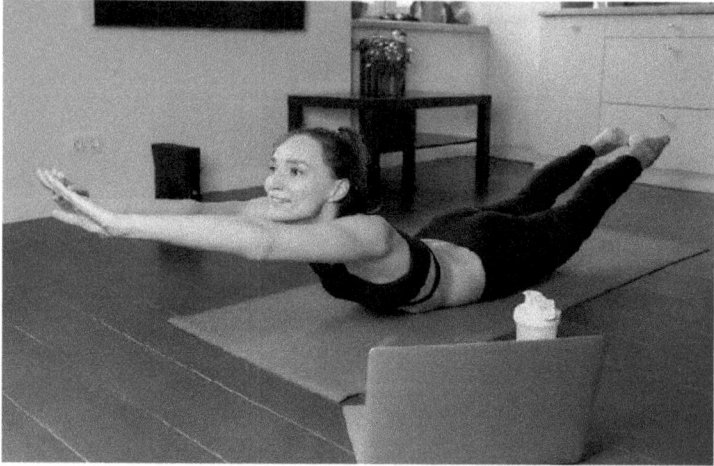

You can also do a variation of the W superman and T superman exercises. In the W-shape variation, squeeze the upper back and bend your arms to form a W-like shape when lifted.

While in the W superman, extend your arms out on either side of your chest to form the T shape.

5. Pull-up superman/prone pull

In a pull-up superman movement, you lie on your chest with your palms on the sides of your chest and in line with your head.

Squeeze your glutes and lower back to enable you to raise your arms and top of the chest a few inches off the floor, and your arms forming the 'W' like shape.

Extend your hands straight out and squeeze your back to pull the arms back to your chest. This movement mimics a pull-up motion. Then extend your arms out again to lower your body and complete one rep.

Get back to the starting position and do more reps before you drop your arms and legs. You can start with a few reps and increase your intensity until you can do three sets of 10 reps.

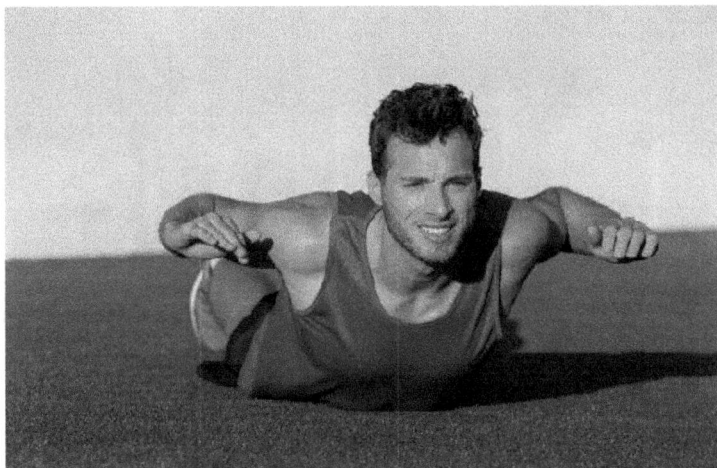

6. Cobra pose

A cobra pose helps you strengthen your ab, back and leg muscles. Start by lying face down with your hands spread on the floor. You can keep your elbows tightly tucked next to your body.

Firmly press your hips and legs on the floor. Straighten your hands while lifting your torso. Hold that position for about 15 to 30 seconds, then go back to the starting position.

Do not strain your elbows or lift higher than you can. Go slowly until you can do three sets of three to five reps simultaneously.

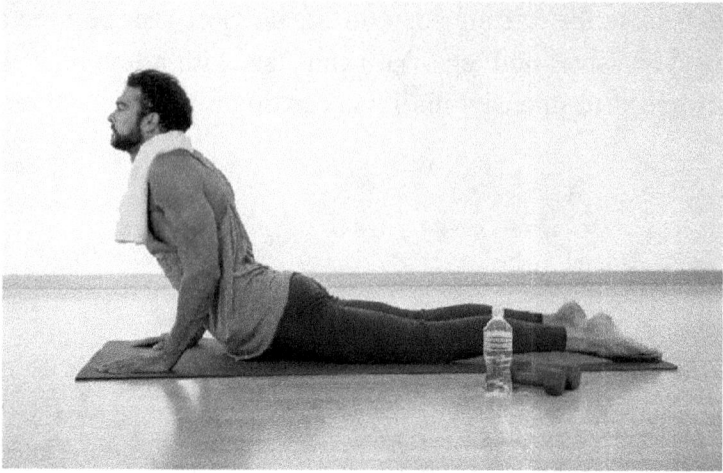

7. Pull-up

In this, grab your pull-up bar with a firm grip with your palms facing forward. Ensure your arms are straight, then pull yourself up the bar until the chest is directly at the bar.

This will help you strengthen your arms then slowly lower yourself down to the starting position. When you lower yourself down, your elbows should be straight, then repeat the same movement for several reps.

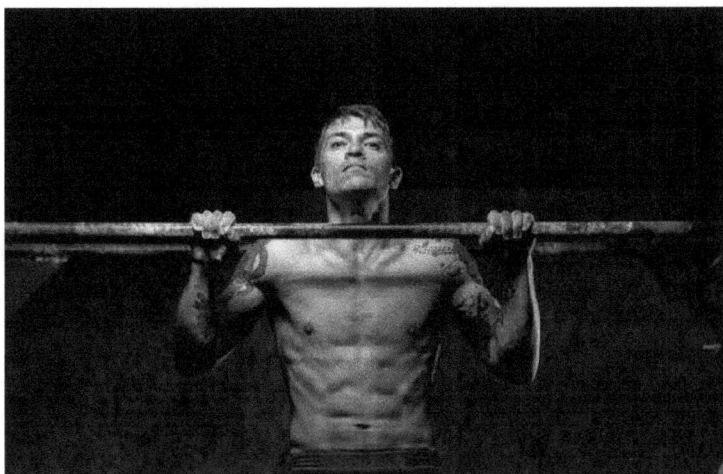

8. T-push-up

In this, you can start either by getting into a push-up or plank position. Place your hands a few inches outside your chest.

Squeeze your core and glutes to ensure your spine is in a straight line. Slightly bend the elbow to push your chest down. At the same time, squeeze your back at the bottom of that movement.

As you push back up to T-shape, squeeze your chest and rotate your body up on one side while raising your other arm straight up at the same time. Hold yourself up at that position, then lower yourself back to the starting position. Repeat the movement on the other side of your body.

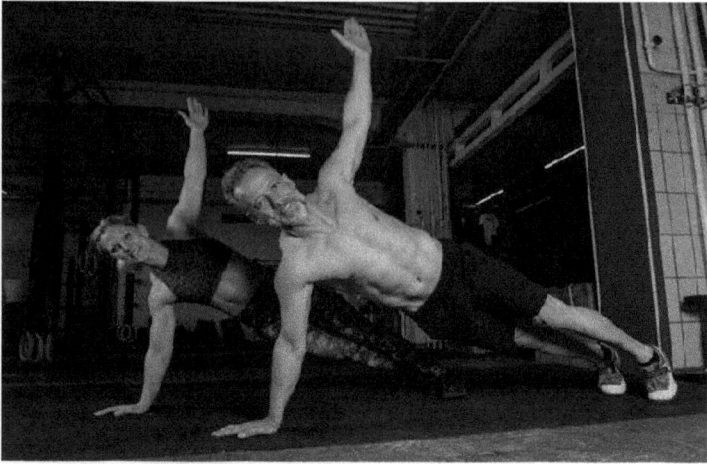

9. Quadruple limb raise

Start by getting into a plank position (on all fours). Ensure your hands are placed shoulder-width apart on the floor. Bend your knee to be directly beneath your hips, and the body parallels to the floor.

Extend your right hand forward and the left leg backward while raised off the floor. Ensure your back is in a straight line from the head to your buttocks. Hold that position for about five to 10 seconds and then lower yourself back to the starting position. Repeat the movement on the other side.

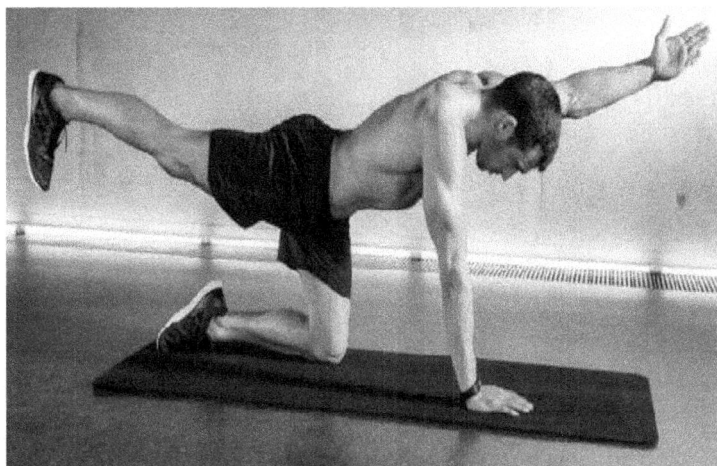

10. Knee-to-chest stretches

Knee-to-chest exercises help to relieve any pain and tension in your lower back. To do this exercise, lie on your back with your head touching the floor.

Keep one foot flat on the floor while bending the knee of the other leg. Use both hands to pull the knee toward your chest. Hold it against the chest for about five seconds. Ensure your abdomen is kept tight and your spine is pressed on the floor.

Lower your leg back to the starting position and do the same with the other leg. You can repeat the movement in each leg two to three times.

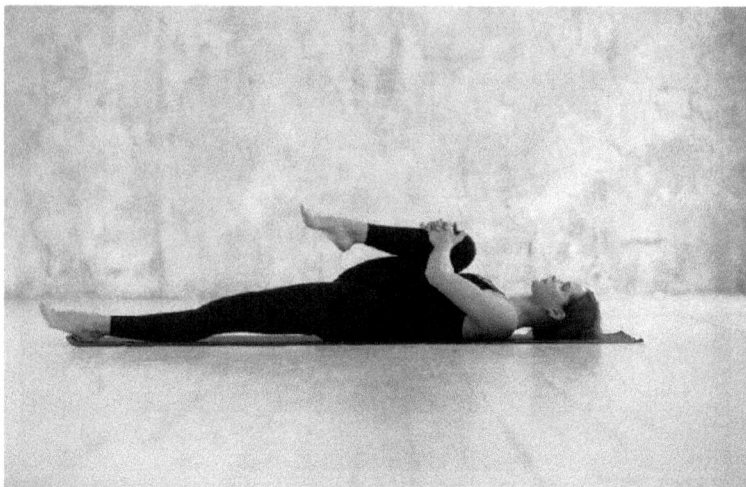

11. Lower back rotational stretch

This is another excellent bodyweight workout that relieves tension on your lower back and works on your core muscles, as well as increases your stability.

Lie back on your yoga mat and bent your knees with your feet placed flat. Keep your shoulders on the floor with your hands spread on your sides to form a T-shape.

Roll your bent knees to one side and hold that position for five to 10 seconds.

Get back to the starting position, roll the bent knees on the opposite side and hold onto that position again. Repeat the movement to work on your lower back and core muscles.

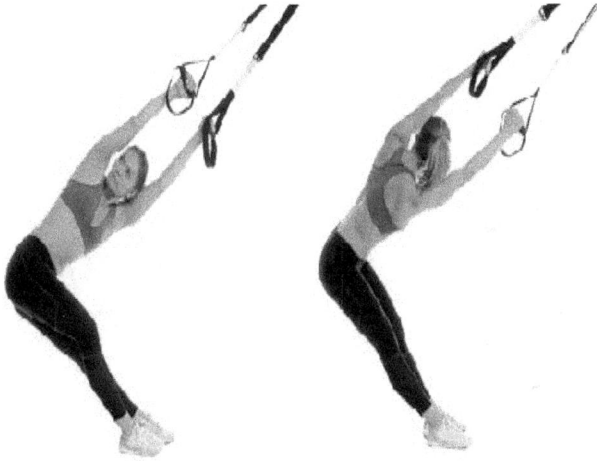

This type of exercise uses a suspension cable. You can do it without the suspension cable and spread your hands on your sides to form the T-shape.

12. Pelvic tilts

Pelvic tilt exercises work on your tight back muscles and make them more flexible. Start by lying on your back on the mat with your knees bent and flat on the surface. Keep the arms to your side and arch your lower back gently. Push out your stomach and hold that position for five seconds.

Flatten your back, then pull your belly button toward the floor and hold that position for five seconds. As you master the move, increase the number of reps you do at a time.

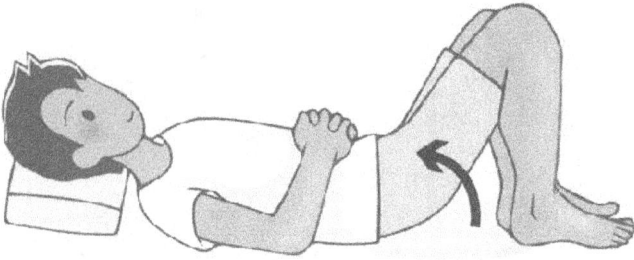

13. Reverse crunch

The reverse crunch is another bodyweight exercise you can use to work on your core muscles. It is excellent for working on your abdomen muscles.

To do this type of exercise, lie down on your back with your face up. Bent your knees at 90° with your feet placed flat on the floor. Keep your arms on your sides with the palms down.

Lift your feet off the floor, raise your thighs until they're vertical, and ensure your knees are still bent at 90°.

Push your knees toward your face, tuck them as far as you can go. Do not lift your mid-back off the floor. Only your lower back and hips should be lifted off the floor.

Hold that position for a few seconds, then lower your feet back until they touch the floor. Repeat the movement until you're able to do 10 to 12 reps. You can start with a single set and increase the sets and reps you do as you get stronger.

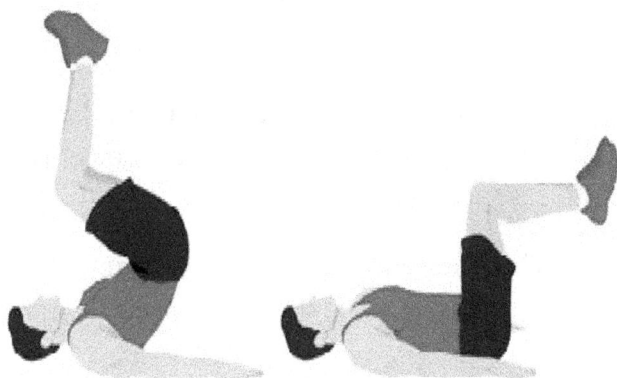

Chapter Summary

Working on your core and back muscles makes you more flexible, prevents injuries, and improves your stability. If you experience back pain often, these types of exercises can help you relieve your condition.

The above exercises are easy to do and are used by both beginners and advanced fitness fanatics. You can begin with a few reps, and as you get stronger, you can increase the number of reps and sets done.

Always make sure you do the exercises correctly. Otherwise, you will be doing more harm than obtaining the desired benefits. If you experience some pain when doing the exercise, you can stop and try it another day. Do not strain your muscles.

Although the exercises can solve various health issues, if you're experiencing severe pain that can't be solved with exercise, please see a doctor.

In the next chapter, you will learn bodyweight exercises to work on your thighs and the large leg muscles.

8

Bodyweight Exercises for Working Thigh Muscles

THIGHS AND LEGS have the largest muscle groups compared to other parts of your body. You can do various bodyweight exercises to target the calves, glutes, hamstrings and quads.

If you're consistent with the workouts, you can notice the changes within a week or two.

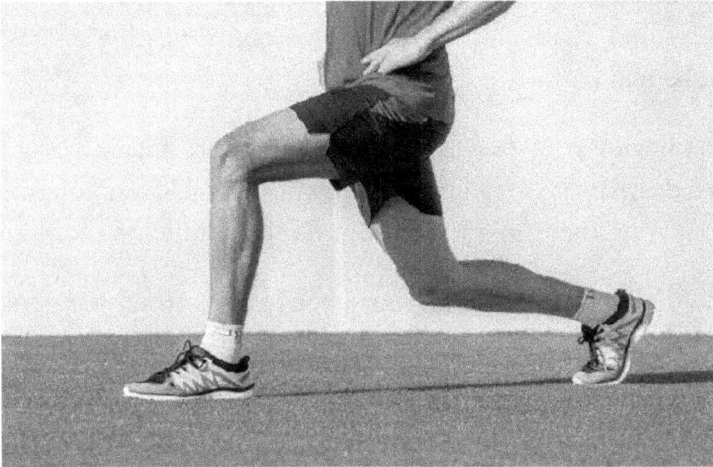

Your thigh has three fascial compartments that house about 18 muscles. These muscles are responsible for your knee's rotation, flexion, extension and abduction of your hips.

Since your thighs have more muscle mass, engaging in various workouts that target thigh muscles will help burn more calories even when sitting down.

Strengthening your thigh muscles makes it easy for you to walk, ride bicycles and even climb stairs. They also help you improve your resting metabolic rate.

The muscles found on your thighs and hips helps you maintain an erect posture and enable rotation of your thighs outward.

Thigh and legs exercises

1. Squats

Squats are one of the best workouts that engage your core, glutes and quads. Squats ensure you have healthy and firm thighs and legs.

Stand with your feet shoulder-width apart and lower your hips down as if you want to sit down. As you lower your hips, bend your knees to 45° and your thighs parallel to the floor.

The depth you can bend your knees varies from one person to the other. This is because the depth depends on one's lower body strength, anatomy and mobility.

Lift yourself and repeat this movement for eight to 10 reps.

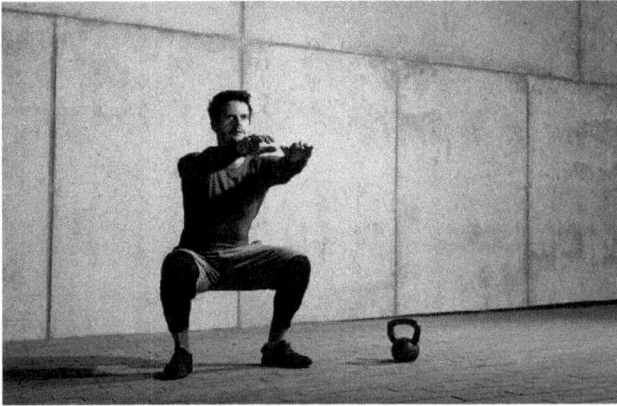

2. Jump squat

Jump squat is a modified squat that increases the intensity of your workout. It works on your fast-twitch muscle fibers found in your legs and increases your heart rate. As a result, you're able to burn more calories.

Just like in a regular squat move, instead of raising to start position slowly, you add an explosive jump to get back straight up, then land softly and quietly to your starting position.

Once you get into a squat position so that your thighs are parallel to the floor, you can then have an explosive jump as high as you can. When landing, you can bend your knees to be at 45°. Get into another squat position and hold there for a second before you jump again.

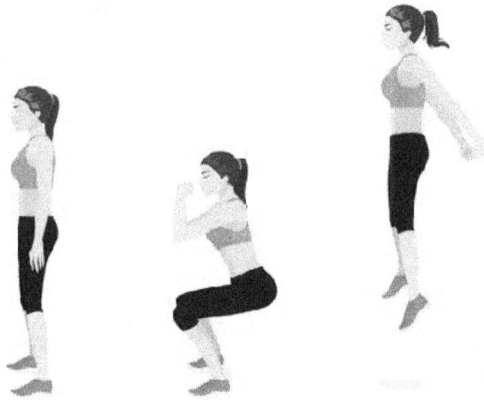

3. Sumo squat

Sumo squat is another variation of squat that engages your hip muscles and works on your quads and glutes. Stand with your feet placed wider apart than shoulder-width. Turn your toes slightly out like a sumo wrestler.

Maintain an upright posture and lower your hips down toward your heels while driving your knees out. When squatting down, make sure your knees are kept behind your toes while the shin is maintained vertically at the bottom of the squat.

Slowly stand up by pushing your heels down and out, then push your hips forward to an extended position.

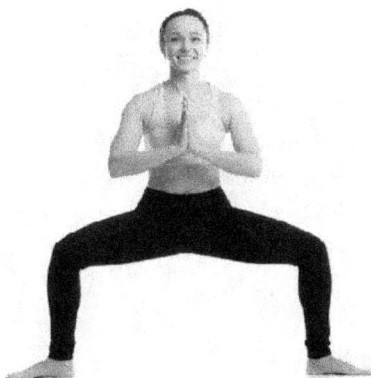

4. Side lunge

Put your feet wide apart (twice shoulder-width apart). Push your hips to the back and the left side. Keep your right leg straight when moving the hips. Bend the left knee, lower your body so that your left thigh is in a parallel position with the floor.

Ensure your feet are flat on the floor when doing the movements. Hold that position for at least two seconds before getting back. Complete reps and switch to the other side.

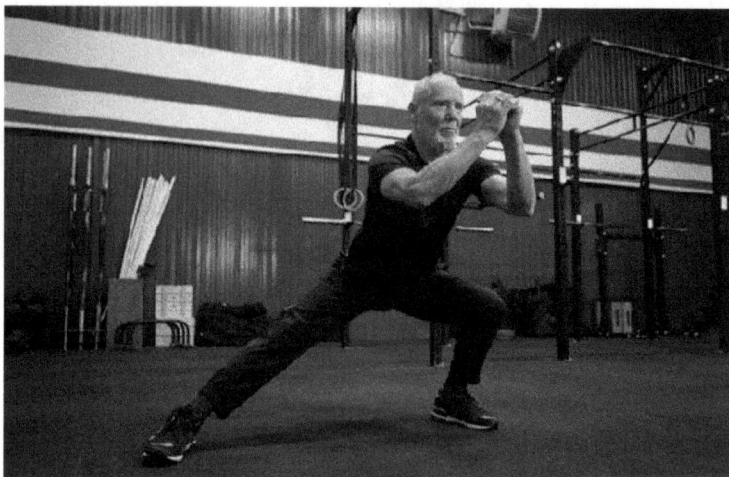

5. Jump lunge

Just like in a jump squat, you can do a jump to a lunge workout. This is an advanced form of lunge exercise, so master the lunge exercise before doing the jump lunge.

Jump lunge works on your fast-twitch muscle fibers that burn fat in your body and increase your heart rate.

To do this exercise, get into a standard lunge position. Once you lower yourself down into lunge position, jump up, then switch your legs so that the opposite leg is at the front when you land. You should land softly and quietly.

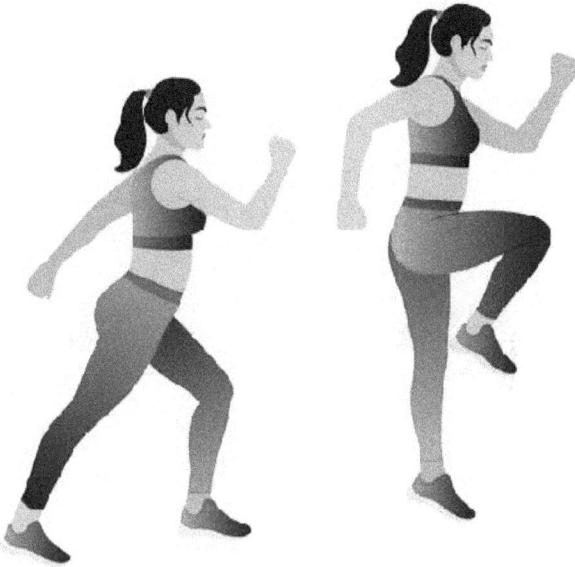

6. Glute bridge

If you have an injury and find it difficult to squat or do a lunge, you can do a glute bridge exercise. This type of bodyweight exercise activates your glutes, hamstrings and lower back muscles.

Lie down on your back with your head touching the floor. Bend your knees and place your feet flat on the floor to about shoulder-width apart. Then raise your hips off the floor while pushing your heels down onto the floor.

Once your hips are higher up, squeeze your glute, and tighten your abdominal muscle. This prevents you from arching your lower back. Keep the shins vertical and hold that position for

251

two seconds, then lower yourself back to the starting position.

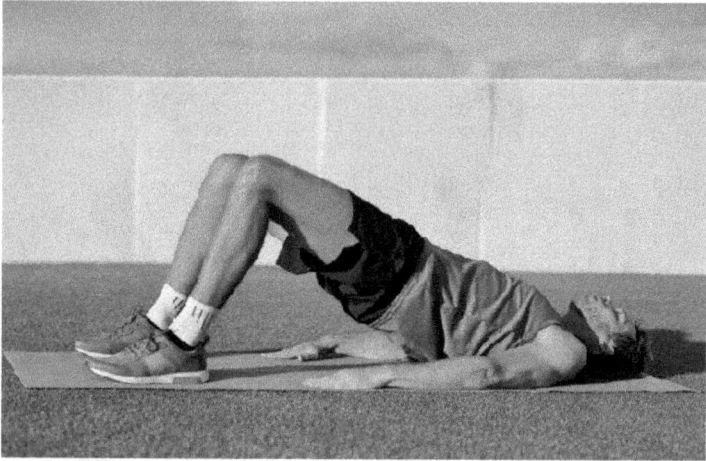

7. Single-leg glute bridge

Lie down face up with your arms out on your sides. Bend your right foot and firmly place the heel of your foot on the ground and extend your left leg to be straight.

Activate your abs and contract your glute muscles to enable you to push your hips up into the bridge position and then lift your left leg off the floor and in line with your right thigh.

While at the top, squeeze glute muscles and then lower yourself back down. Your left leg should be off the floor when doing all reps. Switch legs and repeat the same steps.

You can also use a suspension trainer to increase the intensity of this type of workout.

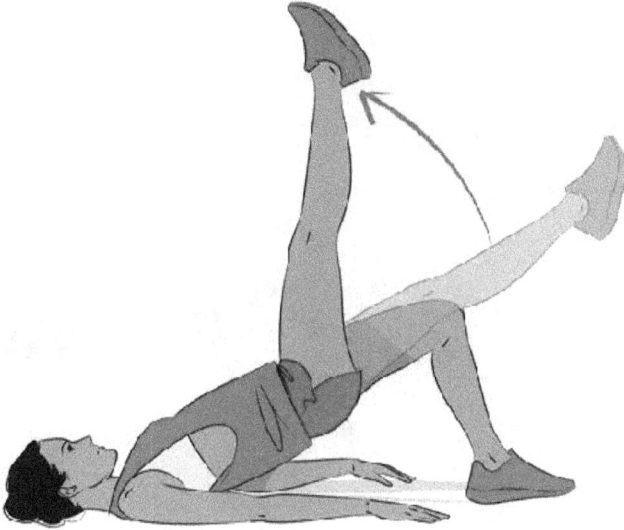

8. Supine leg curl

Lie with your back on the floor, and place your feet on a slippery object like a towel or some socks. Lift your hips off the floor, extend your legs straight forward, and slightly pull your heels back under your body.

This type of exercise puts more pressure on your hamstrings muscles and adds more flexion and extension to your knee. It also works on your glutes and lower back muscles.

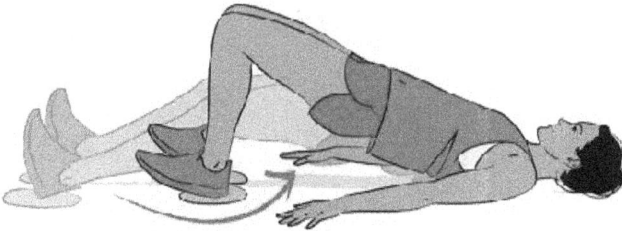

Chapter Summary

Exercising your thigh and leg muscles helps you in correcting any muscle imbalance and injuries. The exercise can also tighten your lower back and strengthen your core.

Including several exercises in your workout routine allow you to focus on a particular group of muscles and improve your overall well-being. Most people tend to neglect their leg muscles and only work out the upper body muscles. But, to have a healthy, balanced, and stable body, you need to include your leg and thigh muscles in your fitness plan.

Be consistent with the exercises because the large leg muscles form an integral part of your fitness goals. Working on this group of muscles keeps your body balanced and makes it easy to work on your upper body muscles. They also help you boost your athletic performance.

Do not overtrain your muscles and balance your exercise routine to focus on both glutes and hamstrings.

Final Words

Bodyweight exercises are essential to build your muscle mass and strengthen your cardiovascular system and nervous system. You don't need any equipment or subscribe to a gym to maintain your fitness goals.

You can do the exercises from anywhere and at any time. You can easily do the exercises in the comfort of your home or even in your office. There are so many reasons why you should include bodyweight exercises in your fitness journey.

These exercises are cost-effective, time-efficient, highly scalable, safe, flexible, and can easily combine cardio and strength training. Strength-training exercises help you increase your body image, improve your body mechanism, boost your energy levels, manage chronic health diseases, burn fat and build lean muscles.

A whole-body workout helps you to be more flexible, effectively lose weight, increase your endurance level, improve your balance, and reduce the risk of injuries and pains.

The exercises rely on your bodyweight to provide you with the resistance needed for the movements. To achieve the desired results, you need to be consistent with the workouts.

If you're looking forward to increasing muscle mass, you have to do the exercises quickly and make the muscles more explosive.

Also, it helps to focus on the strength-training principles to achieve the desired results: Simplicity, individualism, progression and overload. Always focus on a specific type of exercise to work on certain kinds of muscles, especially if you have limited time.

Stick to what works for you. Our bodies are different, so if specific exercises work for your friend, it doesn't mean it will work for you. Start with simple steps. Once your body gets used to the exercises, you can increase your workload, time and resistance. Increasing your workload with the right rest time will result in an overload.

Before starting any exercise, you need to have a warm-up session of at least five to 10 minutes. If you're targeting a specific muscle, do a warm-up to activate those muscles before beginning the actual workout. You should also avoid overtraining to avoid any injuries and exhaustion.

When planning to start your workout routine, you need to check your health and then develop your workout plan. The workout plan helps you determine your fitness level that works as your benchmark to compare your progress.

After knowing your body composition, muscle density and flexibility, you can develop your fitness program. You need to decide your fitness goals, type of exercises to do, and what muscle groups on which to work.

Create a balanced routine to help you achieve your goals. Incorporate the exercises into your daily routine. Include different types of activities, as well as incorporate high-intensity exercises and recovery time. Avoid doing the exercises continuously without any rest. This can result in injuries or joint pains.

Assemble all the tools you need for your exercise. For example, have a yoga mat, a tracking device, sports shoes and others.

Start slow with simple steps and proceed gradually. If you have a busy schedule, you can break down the exercises to have several sessions of exercises per day. You can incorporate several numbers of exercises to do per week. You don't have to limit yourself to a few of them.

Pay more attention to your body. How do you feel after every exercise? If you have been pushing yourself too much, then it's time to slow down and take a break.

Monitor your progress every month to know whether you're on the right track. Can you achieve your fitness goals with the current phase? If not, you should increase your exercise time or intensity of the workout to obtain measurable benefits.

If you didn't achieve your fitness goals, don't give up. Just set up new goals and new exercise activities to do. You can also include your family and friends in the exercises to have more fun.

You should also determine workout days and rest days. You should be consistent to achieve the desired results. Your workout plan should have high-intensity workouts followed by recovery days with light exercises and rest days.

Based on your fitness goals, you can choose the number of sets and reps you're supposed to do on each type of exercise.

After deciding on your workout plan, it is time to start your exercises that target different muscle types. For example, bodyweight exercises that target upper body muscles like your arms muscles.

Exercises that strengthen your arms target your shoulders, biceps and triceps. These exercises engage your core and allow you to work on different muscles simultaneously. You don't need any equipment to do the exercises.

All you need is a proper workout plan and flexing the muscles of your forearms and triceps. Some of the typical bodyweight workouts for arms include dips, tricep dips with lifted legs, pull-ups, chin-ups, plank, up-and-down plank, push-ups, and inchworm with shoulder taps, among others. These exercises not only build muscles but also help you in burning calories.

You also need to work on your neck and shoulder muscles. Neck and shoulders are incredibly mobile, and some motions may leave you with some pain or injuries. Thus, the need to strengthen your neck and shoulder muscles.

Working out your neck and shoulder muscles makes you more flexible and improves your overall body structure. The exercises also help prevent injuries on your delicate areas, such as the shoulder joints.

Shoulder and neck exercises work on your rotator cuff and deltoid muscles. Some of the best exercises you can include in your plan include incline push-up, push-back push-up, plank to down dog, elevated pike push-up, plank up, wall walk, crab walk, reverse burpees, etc.

You can also incorporate neck-stretching exercises to relieve any neck pain and strengthen the neck muscles. Stretching and exercising the neck muscles will improve your posture and leave your head in a neutral position.

Different types of exercises target different neck muscles, including a variety of exercises in your neck workout. This includes exercise, such as chin tuck, prone cobra, and back burn.

Another set of muscles you need to work out is your chest and biceps. These muscles help you improve your physique and stabilize your shoulder joints.

Chest muscles are critical as they support all your daily body functions, acting as the foundation for almost all types of workouts. These muscles control the movement of your arms up, down and across.

Some of the chest workouts you can include in your workout plan include push-up, decline push-up, push-up hold, star plank, chaturanga, dive-bomber push-up, etc.

Some of these chest muscle workouts target your abs, deltoids and triceps. They enable you to get the perfect muscles you need to show off on a beach.

We also discussed various exercises you can use to work out your core and lower back muscles. These exercises help you prevent hunched shoulders and reduce back pains. Choosing the right type of exercise and the number of reps will increase your blood flow and reduce the lower back's stiffness. For better results, you need to engage your abs and back muscles together.

Exercises include the low plank, high-plank, bridge, superman, pull-up, pull-up superman, t-pushup, cobra pose, reverse crunch and pelvic tilt. You can do any of these exercises to reduce any pain and solve various health issues.

To complete your whole-body exercises, you need to work on your thigh and leg muscles. Our legs consist of the largest number of muscles and have more muscle mass.

Most of the leg workouts target your calves, glutes, hamstrings and quads. Exercises that target these different muscles help you burn more calories and improve your metabolic rate.

Exercising your thigh and leg muscles regularly enables you to tone your muscles and ensure you have strong thighs and legs. The best workouts for your legs muscles include squats, jump squats, sumo squats, side lunge, jump lunge, glute-bridge and supine leg curl.

For effective results, you have to include both simple and high intensive exercises. You can also increase the number of reps you do in each workout once you master the move. Adding some variations to the exercises enables you to increase your heart rate.

Remember to do a warm-up before beginning the exercises and some stretches after the exercises to increase your body's blood flow. Choosing the right type of activity and a proper diet will help you achieve your fitness goals.

Author's Note

I hope you enjoy this book as much as I loved writing it. If you do, it would be wonderful if you could take a short minute and leave a review on **Amazon** as soon as you can, as your kind feedback is much appreciated and so very important.

Thank you!

References

https://en.wikipedia.org/wiki/Calisthenics

https://www.mensjournal.com/health-fitness/how-to-build-muscle-without-lifting-weights/

https://www.ownyoureating.com/blog/10-reasons-why-bodyweight-training-is-the-best-form-of-exercise/

https://www.realbuzz.com/articles-interests/fitness/article/the-four-principles-of-training/

https://www.womenshealthmag.com/fitness/a30522035/what-is-strength-training/

https://www.healthline.com/health/fitness-nutrition/no-weight-workout

https://www.verywellfit.com/complete-beginners-guide-to-strength-training-1229585

https://www.healthline.com/nutrition/how-to-start-exercising#TOC_TITLE_HDR_5

https://www.mayoclinic.org/healthy-lifestyle/fitness/in-depth/fitness/art-20048269

https://www.nerdfitness.com/blog/how-to-build-your-own-workout-routine/

https://www.nerdfitness.com/blog/beginner-body-weight-workout-burn-fat-build-muscle/

https://www.mensjournal.com/health-fitness/9-best-bodyweight-moves-develop-colossal-arms/3-suspension-trainer-biceps-curls/

https://greatist.com/fitness/bodyweight-workout-for-biceps#beginner

https://www.menshealth.com/fitness/a25620352/best-bodyweight-back-exercises/

https://www.mensjournal.com/health-fitness/best-bodyweight-exercises-legs/15-swiss-ball-wall-squat/

Resistance Band Exercises for Seniors Over 50
By Francis Papun
© Copyright 2023 Francis Papun

www.ingramcontent.com/pod-product-compliance
Lightning Source LLC
Chambersburg PA
CBHW070100030426
42335CB00016B/1959